Praise for
Tell Me What to Eat If I Am Trying to Conceive

"Tell Me What To Eat If I Am Trying To Conceive *is full of sensible advice and fabulous tips for eating well—and all from a true nutrition expert! It's a practical, common-sense guide for any woman who wants to take better care of her body."*

—Dana Angelo White, MS, RD, ATC

Tell Me What to Eat If I Am Trying to Conceive

Nutrition You Can Live With

By Kimberly A. Tessmer, RD, LD

Foreword by Elaine Magee

NEW PAGE BOOKS
A division of The Career Press, Inc.
Pompton Plains, NJ

Tell Me What to Eat If I Am Trying to Conceive
Edited and Typeset by Kathryn Henches
Cover design by Lucia Rossman/Digi Dog Design
Printed in the U.S.A.

To order this title, please call toll-free 1-800-CAREER-1 (NJ and Canada: 201-848-0310) to order using VISA or MasterCard, or for further information on books from Career Press.

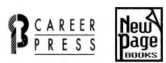

The Career Press, Inc.
220 West Parkway, Unit 12
Pompton Plains, NJ 07444

www.careerpress.com
www.newpagebooks.com

Library of Congress Cataloging-in-Publication Data

Tessmer, Kimberly A.

Tell me what to eat if I am trying to conceive : nutrition you can live with / by Kimberly A. Tessmer ; foreword by Elaine Magee.

      p. cm.

Includes bibliographical references and index.

ISBN 978-1-60163-171-8 -- ISBN 978-1-60163-655-3 (ebook) 1. Infertility, Female--Diet therapy--Popular works. 2. Infertility, Female--Nutritional aspects--Popular works. I. Title.

RG201.T47 2011

618.1'780654--dc22   2011003526

Dedication

I know all too well the emotional and at times frustrating journey of trying to conceive, and so I dedicate this book to my little girl, Tori, who made it all worthwhile. She is the light of our lives and I don't know what we would do without her. I'd also like to dedicate this book to my Dad and my late Mom, whom I miss dearly. They taught me that anything is possible and showed me that parenthood is precious.

Acknowledgments

I would like to sincerely thank all of the health professionals who offered their advice, recommendations, and delicious recipes for this book. Thank you also to *all* of my family and friends for your love, support, and encouragement—particularly my wonderful husband, Greg, who is always by my side and supports me in all my endeavors.

Contents

Chapter 2:
Weighing in on Your Fertility
47

Chapter 3:
Diet Rules to Eat By
69

Chapter 4:
Everything You Always Wanted
to Ask a Dietitian About Trying to Conceive
93

Chapter 5:
Conception-Welcoming Nutrients
for Her and Him
111

Chapter 6:
Fertility-Friendly Alternative Therapies
131

Chapter 7:
Navigating Unproven Diet Remedies
147

Chapter 8:
Help Boost Your Chances With
Delicious Recipes and Meal Plans
155

Resources
183

Bibliography
193

Index
199

About the Author
205

Disclaimer

At the time this book was written all information in this book was believed by the author to be correct and accurate. Information on trying to conceive changes frequently as more research is being completed. Always keep yourself up-to-date by reading reputable and current publications and speaking with your healthcare provider. The author shall have no liability of any kind for damages of any nature, however caused. The author will not accept any responsibility for any omissions, misinterpretations, or misstatements that may exist within this book. The author does not endorse any product or company listed in this book. Always consult with your healthcare provider for medical advice as well as recommendations on any type of supplement or herbal supplement you plan on taking while trying to conceive. The author is not engaged in rendering medical services and this book should not be construed as medical advice nor should it take the place of regular scheduled appointments with your healthcare provider and dietitian on a regular basis.

Foreword

For some couples, getting pregnant and staying pregnant comes easily. For other couples, it can be the most trying time of their lives. But I believe information is power and I hope it will bring you hope, as well. Reading this book will give you essential information concerning conception whether you are underweight and over exercising or the opposite.

Registered dietitian Kimberly Tessmer navigates you through a variety of medical conditions that are potentially not conducive to conception—from PCOS to celiac disease. Throughout the book you will find answers to all of your specific food and beverage questions about what to limit if you're trying to become pregnant, and why (from coffee, soft drinks, and alcohol to soy food, vitamin supplements, and a vegetarian diet).

According to the American Society for Reproductive Medicine, if you don't get pregnant after 12 months of regular unprotected intercourse—or six months if you are a woman over 35—it's time to seek help from a fertility specialist. This book will be helpful before and after you and your spouse might come to this point. And speaking of your spouse, this book is an equal opportunity fertility guide, with suggestions for your spouse throughout, including specific precautions (don't smoke) and suggestions on how his nutrient intake may play a role in conception—foods rich in antioxidant vitamins C and E, and the minerals selenium and zinc, for example, may improve sperm count and/or the ability of sperm to reach the egg.

But it's not all about vitamins and minerals—it just may be omega-3s to the rescue once again. No matter what I write about, it seems—even diet and fertility—omega-3s are suspected of being beneficial. A recent study on male turkeys, for example, found that a higher ratio of omega-3 to omega-6 fatty acids seemed to help sustain reproductive capacity, especially as they got older (from *Theriogenology,* Jan. 15, 2004, vol. 61 #2, pages 537–549).

Getting some omega-3-s from fish and certain plant foods works for the mom-to-be, as well. Researchers now suspect that the fish omega-3s play a critical role in the development and maintenance of the developing baby's brain and nerve system and might lower the risk for postpartum depression for mom after the birth, as well. (This research was presented on April 12, 2011 at the Experimental Biology meeting in Washington, D.C.)

When it comes to fertility, the "right" weight appears to be "normal weight," with obese, underweight, and extremely lean women tending to have more difficulties getting pregnant (from the *American Journal of Clinical Nutrition*, October, 2008, vol. 88 #4, pages 886–893). Kimberly Tessmer devotes an entire chapter to this.

Living and eating healthfully (and with low stress) and striving for normal body weight are the basic keys to fertility success, but there does appear to be a possible group of "fertility foods" that may improve conception odds, according to a study of 17,000 women, conducted by the Harvard School of Public Health. Including:

- Eat more monounsaturated fats (like olive oil) and fewer trans fats.

- Reduce animal protein (red meat) if excessive in your diet, and increase vegetable protein (like soy).

- Moderate consumption of high-fat diary products like cheese, whole milk, and ice cream.

- Eat more high-fiber, phytochemical-rich carbohydrates (whole grains, beans, vegetables, and fruits) while eating less refined and processed carbohydrates and sugars.

- Avoid alcohol consumption (for women) and excessive alcohol (for men)—it can impair ovulation and sperm production.

With such a critical and emotional topic, it is hard to know what's true and what sensible steps should be taken. You are in great hands with Kimberly. She shares her wisdom (and recipes) on all things related to fertility—from her diet rules to eat by and tips on trying to conceive to alternative therapies.

Let this book guide the way to improved health and a happy pregnancy.

Elaine Magee, MPH, RD

Introduction

With more than 4 million babies being born per year in the United States, it is a good guess that there is a sizeable number of couples trying to conceive at any given time. The leap into the world of trying to conceive can be an exciting one for couples. For some it seems to come easy, yet for others the journey can become difficult and frustrating. When you are trying to get pregnant with no success, it can seem as though everyone around you is getting pregnant accidentally. Although it may seem accidental, it actually requires countless factors lining up just right to make it happen. Your best bet is to go into the trying to conceive (TTC) process knowing it may take some time, so that if it doesn't happen right away you'll be able to hang in there longer without getting too frustrated. If it happens sooner, then it is all that more of a wonderful surprise!

To start the process of TTC off on the right foot, it is important to know that your diet and lifestyle are two very important factors that will help improve your fertility naturally. In fact, new research is making the connection between diet and fertility even more apparent. A well-balanced diet helps to regulate the body's hormones and properly nourish your reproductive system. A healthy weight and active lifestyle can also greatly impact a woman's as well as a man's fertility. The key to improving your chances of becoming pregnant is to know your body, focus on what you put in it, keep it as healthy as possible, and understand your individual fertility cycle. Your body will provide you with signs and signals every cycle, which will help guide you to success. But it is up to *you* to take care of some of the rest, and this book is meant to help guide you through some of the process.

You may find it interesting to know that although the odds of conception vary greatly from couple to couple, depending on factors such as age, weight, and health status, in general couples have just about a 25-percent chance of becoming pregnant each cycle. The good news is that after five to six months, that percentage goes up to about 50 percent, and after one year, most couples have about an 85-percent chance of becoming pregnant. The sooner you start to take care of your body—and that goes for both women and men—the more likely you are to achieve success. If you have picked this book up to read, you already realize that diet and health definitely have a strong influence on your ability to conceive, and that is a positive first step.

It can take as long as 12 to 18 months of trying before a couple becomes pregnant; most physicians will not intervene before 12 months unless there is a history of fertility issues that would result in the couple not being able to become pregnant on their own. So for many couples, if they do not become pregnant right away, they could be on their own for up to 12 months. During those months it is good to have tools at your disposal that will help you to feel empowered and help the process along. This book is meant to provide you with the tools and knowledge you need to have the best chance of becoming pregnant. This book contains the vital information you need to put you on the road to a common-sense approach to eating healthily and living a healthy lifestyle. It will give you the tools to begin achieving a healthy weight, gearing your body up with the right vitamins, minerals, and antioxidants and relieving your stress. You will also find current information on popular herbs and supplements, as well as some delicious recipes and simple menu plans to get you started on the right foot and keep you on track.

Unfortunately, this book can't guarantee you a pregnancy but it can help set the stage for good health and a healthy pregnancy when it does come along. It will provide you with a foundation for a healthy way of eating for motherhood and beyond and that is a winning combination. This book should not be seen as a substitute for regular visits to your OB/GYN and/or fertility specialist. Instead, it should be used as a complement to your medical team's instructions and advice, and as a reference when needed.

Chapter 1

What You Should Know About Your Fertility and What May Cause Challenges

The best way to tackle any issue is to start at the beginning. Whether you are just beginning your journey to trying to conceive or are already a seasoned veteran, it is a good idea to get back to the basics. This first chapter will aim to answer some general questions concerning fertility and briefly discuss possible challenges to fertility before jumping into the main concept of this book, which is the food and diet aspect of trying to conceive.

? What are the general phases of conception?

Chances are you already know all about the birds and the bees, but do you really know the medical science behind creating a baby? Before you begin your journey of conception, take a moment to understand the incredible process of conception. You will begin to understand just what a miracle babies truly are.

There are three steps your body needs to follow to make a baby: ovulation, fertilization, and implantation. Seems so simple, right?

Well, when you realize the timing that goes into each step and the problems that can happen with each step you can understand why every woman in her early 20s to mid-30s has only a 15- to 25-percent chance of becoming pregnant each month. Unfortunately that percentage dips as a woman ages.

In the first phase, which is ovulation, an immature egg, or *follicle*, develops into a mature egg and is released from one of your ovaries. This egg is available for fertilization for only 12 to 24 hours after it is released. Sperm, on the other hand, can survive for up to 72 hours. If a released egg has not met its sperm within that 12- to 24-hour window of opportunity, the conception window is closed for the month. Ovulation can occur at different times, depending on the individual woman, but typically it happens around two weeks prior to the start of the menstrual cycle. Being able to pinpoint when you will ovulate is the key to planning conception. In the second phase of conception, which is the fertilization phase, there is no time for dinner and a movie! With any luck, a male sperm is quickly introduced and enters the egg. It is at that very moment that the genetic makeup of the baby is already being determined, including the gender of the baby. Within about 24 hours after fertilization, the third and final phase of conception, implantation, takes place. Once an egg is fertilized it will begin dividing and travel through the fallopian tubes into the uterus. At this point your body will begin to produce certain hormones that will help the egg attach to your uterus. One of these hormones is HCG, commonly called the pregnancy hormone, which will turn your home pregnancy test positive. Some women will experience light spotting or bleeding as the egg attaches to the uterus, which is known as *implantation bleeding.*

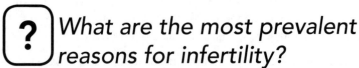 # What are the most prevalent reasons for infertility?

Now we know what needs to happen to make a baby. So what are some of the reasons, besides bad timing, that it does not always happen as planned. First things first. Let's understand what is meant by "fertility" and "infertility" and why they are important to talk about. Your fertility is your natural ability to conceive or become pregnant. Infertility is defined as the inability to become pregnant under the age of 35 after a year of trying to conceive. It can be a problem with the female, the male, or both. Keep in mind that infertility hardly means you will never become pregnant; it only means there might be an underlying reason that needs to be addressed and treated. There is also "unexplained fertility," which means no definitive reason for infertility has been found after all medical tests are performed. Again, this doesn't mean pregnancy cannot occur. The reason it is important to talk about infertility in this book is because this book will focus mainly on diet and nutrition for conception, and for some couples, poor nutrition can be a large part of the problem when it comes to infertility, or not being able to become pregnant. In addition, for some women who deal with infertility due to a specific health-related concern such as PCOS or celiac disease, diet can be a large part of the treatment that will result in finally becoming pregnant.

There are many barriers that can make having a baby challenging. They range from medical issues to lifestyle to everything in between. These problems are associated with the female, the male, or both. Many times there is more then one barrier that may be causing problems, including:

- Not ovulating or poor egg quality
- Absent or irregular periods
- Hormonal imbalances
- Fallopian tube issues
- Pre-existing health issues
- Cancer treatments such as chemotherapy and radiation
- Age (for both female and male)

- Over- or underweight
- Sedentary lifestyle/lack of exercise
- The use of alcohol, drugs, and tobacco.
- Poor diet and nutrition
- Excessive caffeine intake
- Chronic stress
- Lack of proper sleep
- History of STDs (sexually transmitted diseases).
- Male factor issues such as low sperm count or poor

  quality sperm

? When should I seek medical advice?

Keeping the definition of infertility in mind, if you are younger then age 35 and have been unable to conceive after a year of trying, or if you are older than age of 35 and have not been successful at conceiving after six months, it is time to make a visit to your healthcare provider. There could be underlying reasons, some mentioned previously, that are hindering your efforts. Your healthcare provider can perform necessary tests to help better pinpoint the problem(s).

Aside from this rule of thumb, if you have irregular or absent menstrual cycles, known problems with your menstrual cycles and/or ovulation, have experienced multiple miscarriages, have prior use of birth control pills or devices, known health issues, or anything that seems out of the ordinary to you and your body, you may be wise to see your healthcare provider before that time frame. Before you begin your journey of trying to conceive, it is always a good idea to have a complete health check-up with both your primary care physician and your OB/GYN to ensure that everything is in good working order and that you have any health issues and/or medications that can effect both fertility and pregnancy under control.

? What health issues can affect my fertility?

There are many health issues as well as both over-the-counter and prescription medications that can affect your fertility and make it more difficult to conceive. This is why it is vital to visit your healthcare provider before trying to conceive. Some health issues for women include, but are not limited to: uterine fibroids, ovarian cysts, PCOS (polycystic ovary syndrome), and endometriosis. Other health problems that can affect both men and women might include celiac disease, uncontrolled thyroid disorders, and diabetes just to name a few.

? What is PCOS and how can it affect my fertility?

PCOS stands for polycystic ovary (or ovarian) syndrome. It may be a shock to learn that PCOS is one of the most common causes of female infertility. In fact, many women don't even realize they have PCOS until they seek medical help after not being able to become pregnant. PCOS is a condition in which small cysts grow on the ovaries which, in turn, leads to hormone imbalances. It is not the cysts per se that cause the majority of the problems, but the imbalance of hormones. Hormones are what help drive the conception cycle, including the normal development of eggs inside the ovaries. In women with PCOS, eggs do not mature and instead form into ovarian cysts. Ovulation does not occur, and a hormone called *progesterone* is not produced. Without progesterone, the menstrual cycle can be irregular or absent altogether. With PCOS the immature eggs and inability to ovulate is usually caused by low levels of FSH, or *follicle stimulating hormone*, along with higher-than-normal levels of the male hormone (which females also produce) called *androgen*, which is produced in the ovaries. Without mature eggs in the ovaries, conception cannot occur and infertility is the result.

Still another hormone greatly affected by PCOS is *insulin*. Insulin is a hormone that helps to regulate blood sugar levels in the body. Many women with PCOS experience high blood sugar levels because their bodies are ineffective at utilizing insulin and, therefore, regulating glucose or blood sugar. This is called *insulin resistance*. Over time, insulin resistance can increase the risk for diabetes. In addition, excess insulin also appears to increase the production of androgen, again causing hormonal imbalance. Besides infertility and insulin resistance, hormonal imbalances can also lead to:

- Heavy, irregular, or absent menstrual cycles
- Worsening acne and other skin problems
- Increased body and facial hair
- Thinning hair on the scalp
- Weight gain and/or obesity, with trouble losing weight
- Depression and/or anxiety

FYI: The cause of PCOS is yet unknown; however, it is believed that genetics can play a role. It is estimated that as many as 5 million women of childbearing age in the United States are afflicted with PCOS.

At present, there is no cure for PCOS. It is important to diagnose it early and to manage it in order to minimize symptoms as well as health problems later in life such as type 2 diabetes, heart disease, hypertension (high blood pressure), and uterine cancer. Treatment goals are based on the woman's individual symptoms, future health, and whether or not she trying to conceive. Many women need a combination of treatments to reach their goals. Although PCOS is not curable, the good news is that there are treatments that can help to manage and alleviate symptoms such as lifestyle modification (including a healthy diet, exercise, and weight loss), birth control pills to help control hormone levels and regulate menstrual cycles, insulin lowering medications, and androgen lowering medications.

Dietary management is an essential part of the treatment and care of PCOS.

Research has suggested that some of the following dietary recommendations can be beneficial for most women with PCOS:

- Choose foods that are lower in saturated fats, such as lean meats, fish, and low-fat or fat-free dairy products, and increase your intake of healthy unsaturated fats (monounsaturated and polyunsaturated) such as olive oil, fish, nuts, and avocados.

- Choose a diet high in fiber including fruits, vegetables, whole grains, nuts, and seeds.

- Limit refined carbohydrates such as processed foods that include added sugars and white flours and choose complex carbohydrates more often, such as whole-grain breads, brown rice, whole-grain pasta, whole-grain cereals, oatmeal, nuts, fruits, and vegetables.

- Pay attention to *all* serving sizes but especially carbohydrate serving sizes. They should usually be much smaller then you think.

- Choose foods with a lower glycemic index or, better yet, a lower glycemic load.

- Eat often, at least every 3 to 4 hours.

- Include a lean protein along with a low glycemic or whole-grain carbohydrate or healthy fat with all meals and snacks to help manage blood sugar levels.

FYI: In general, glycemic index and glycemic load provide information on how a specific food affects blood sugar and insulin levels. In other words, they can help us figure out which foods are good and bad for helping to better control blood sugar levels. Glycemic index (GI) is a numerical system that measures how much the carbohydrate in a particular food increases blood sugar after it is consumed. The higher the number or GI, the greater the spike in blood sugar. A food with a low GI will cause a smaller rise in blood sugar. However there can be some shortfalls to this system. Glycemic load (GL) can be a better indicator because it also takes into account how much of that carbohydrate is in a standard serving of a particular food. For example, the carbohydrate in watermelon has a high GI, but there isn't much of it in a standard serving so it has a relatively low GL. Foods that have a low GL usually have a low GI. Foods with a moderate to high GL can range from very low to very high GI.

Regular moderate physical activity is also encouraged to help manage blood sugar levels, body weight, and stress levels. Women with PCOS who are overweight should be encouraged to reach a healthy weight in a smart way by losing weight slowly and steadily with a healthy diet approach, appropriate portion sizes, and plenty of regular moderate physical activity. In addition, your healthcare provider and/or dietitian may recommend a multivitamin/mineral supplement, additional vitamin D, calcium, fish oil, and other supplements. Always speak with your healthcare provider first before beginning any supplemental intake or embarking on any weight loss and/or exercise program.

If you are having fertility problems and notice some of the symptoms mentioned previously, you should see your healthcare provider to be properly diagnosed. If you have already been diagnosed with PCOS, it is vital that you get your symptoms under control so that conception is possible and so that you reduce your risk of other related health problems in the future. Talk to your healthcare provider about treating all of your symptoms, not just the ones that deal with trying to conceive. Speak to a registered dietitian that specializes in PCOS who can properly guide you with the key dietary treatments of PCOS including diet, exercise, and weight loss. At the end of this book you will find valuable resources that can provide you with more information on PCOS.

(?) *What is endometriosis and how can it affect my fertility?*

Endometriosis is commonly diagnosed in women of childbearing age. It is a condition that causes the tissue that normally lines the inside of the uterus (called *endometrium*) to grow in areas outside the uterus, usually in the pelvic region. Each month, the body releases hormones whose job it is to thicken the endometrium and get ready to nest a possible fertilized egg. If there is no fertilized egg, the endometrium breaks down and the body eliminates it as blood, which is the menstrual cycle. With endometriosis, the tissue that finds its way outside of the uterus acts just like the tissue that lines the inside of the uterus by thickening, breaking down, and bleeding. However, unlike the tissue inside the uterus, the tissue outside of the uterus has no way of being eliminated by the body so it becomes trapped. Surrounding tissue usually becomes irritated and eventually forms scar tissue and cysts. This whole process can cause pelvic pain, sometimes severe, along with heavy periods, bleeding between periods, pain with bowel movements or urination, and infertility. Other symptoms that may present themselves can include fatigue, diarrhea, constipation, nausea, and bloating. Endometriosis can be classified as mild, moderate, or severe. Some women can experience severe symptoms, whereas others may not even know they have the condition until they realize they are having problems becoming pregnant and go in to see their healthcare provider. Usually, women with moderate to severe endometriosis tend to have more difficulty becoming pregnant than those women with milder cases.

A balanced diet is important for all of us because it can help improve our overall health. For women with endometriosis, a healthy and well-balanced diet can also be a benefit by increasing their ability to tolerate medical treatments and better deal with potential side effects. A registered dietitian who specializes in women's health issues can help put together an appropriate dietary plan for women affected by endometriosis.

At present there is no known cause or cure for endometriosis, but there are successful treatments. The key is early diagnosis, which can help to reduce unnecessary complications and pain. A woman's treatment plan depends on her own individual needs, symptoms, age, and conception plans. She should work closely with her physician so that together they can determine the plan that will benefit her most. If you have experienced any of the symptoms mentioned previously, speak with your healthcare provider. The Resources section at the back of this book contains valuable resources that can provide you with more information on endometriosis.

? What is celiac disease and how can it affect my fertility?

Chances are you have probably heard of celiac disease or at the least a gluten-free diet. You have probably heard about it on the news or have spotted the term "gluten-free" on food labels at the store. To give you an idea of how prevalent celiac disease is, recent studies indicate that more then 2 million Americans, or about one out of every 133 people, have the disease. The biggest dilemma is that at this point, not enough people are properly diagnosed and if they are diagnosed, it can take up to several years or more to get to that point. This is harsh for anyone experiencing the symptoms that untreated and/or undiagnosed or even misdiagnosed celiac disease can cause. For women who are trying to become pregnant and are experiencing infertility due to undiagnosed celiac disease, this can drastically shorten their reproductive years and can be quite frustrating. Many health professionals feel that all women with infertility issues should be tested for celiac disease for just this reason. The good news is that the rate at which adults are being diagnosed is increasing rapidly thanks to greater awareness and knowledge and improved technology. If your physician suspects celiac disease, you should be referred to a gastroenterologist (a specialist in the areas of the stomach and intestines) who has expertise in this disease. The first step in the diagnosis process is a simple blood test to screen for certain antibodies in the blood. If the blood test comes back positive, that indicates that you will need further evaluation, specifically a biopsy of the lining of the small intestines. This is the gold standard to proper diagnosis of celiac disease.

What does celiac disease have to do with fertility? Let's start with what exactly celiac disease is. Celiac disease is an autoimmune inflammatory disorder of the small intestine. It is a disease that can affect men and women as well as children, and most likely has some type of genetic link. In fact, in many cases, women with infertility issues are not properly diagnosed until a family member is diagnosed and a link is made. For people who have been diagnosed with celiac disease, consuming any food or beverage that contains gluten causes their body to produce specific antibodies that attack the small intestine. These antibodies destroy the *villi* (hairs) within the lining of the small intestine as well as digestive enzymes. Once the villi in the small intestine are destroyed, the body loses its ability to absorb nutrients needed for good health, such as carbohydrates, protein, fat, vitamins, minerals, and other essential disease-fighting phytonutrients.

These nutritional deficiencies, along with the destruction of the lining of the small intestine, can lead to a long list of serious health problems and symptoms that can include infertility, not only in women but also in men. Even if a woman with undiagnosed celiac disease is able to become pregnant, there is a higher risk of miscarriage, and if the fetus survives, there can be problems for both the mother and baby if the mother has not been diagnosed and treated. The key is for women to be diagnosed and treated before conception occurs. Even if a woman eliminates gluten from her diet, she should wait a certain amount of time, depending on her physician's recommendation, for the villi in the small intestine to heal and absorb nutrients properly before attempting conception.

Some people can be asymptomatic for years until something triggers the disease, such as surgery, viral infection, severe emotional stress, pregnancy, and/or childbirth. Not only does celiac disease cause a myriad of concerns and symptoms of the gastrointestinal tract, but it has been found that it can affect just about every system in the body, including the neurological, endocrine, orthopedic, hematological, and reproductive systems. Both children and adults can experience one or more of the following symptoms:

- Reoccurring abdominal bloating and pain
- Pale and foul-smelling stool
- Depression
- Nausea and vomiting
- Bone or joint pain
- Diarrhea
- Muscle cramps
- Weight loss
- Constipation
- Iron deficiency with or without unexplained anemia
- Chronic alternating diarrhea with constipation
- Excessive flatulence
- Known vitamin and mineral deficiencies
- Balance problems
- Migraines

- Edema or excessive fluid retention
- Seizures or other neurological reactions
- Chronic fatigue, weakness, and lack of energy
- Memory problems
- Lactose intolerance

Infants and children may also display additional symptoms:

- Failure to thrive
- Growth and maturation problems
- Bloated abdomens
- Learning challenges and disabilities
- Behavioral changes, including irritability
- Dental enamel defects

Once someone with celiac disease begins a gluten-free diet, the tissues of the small intestine begin to heal and the associated symptoms begin to diminish. However, just because the intestine heals doesn't mean they can stop following a gluten-free diet. Any ingestion of gluten will start the destruction all over again, so a gluten-free diet needs to be followed closely for a lifetime.

So what is this gluten in food that wreaks such havoc on people with celiac disease? Gluten is a protein found in wheat, rye, barley, and any derivative of these grains. At one time, oats were also considered to be harmful to people with celiac disease, but recent scientific studies have shown otherwise (when the oats are in pure form). Just like any other diet, a gluten-free diet can be healthy or unhealthy. It depends on the choices one makes. Many of the gluten-free products on the market today can lack nutrients such as iron, B vitamins, and fiber. so you need to learn to make good choices and balance your diet appropriately, just as you would with any other diet. The main focus should still be to eat well-balanced meals and to eat from *all* of the food groups each day. The key is to build your healthy eating plan using alternative grains, and to do that you need to start with the proper education. You must read labels before you eat any food and become skilled at doing so! If the food contains an ingredient that is questionable, avoid the food until you can learn more about it. While you are learning about the foods you can and cannot eat, it is best to stick with foods that are naturally gluten-free, such as plain poultry, fish, and meats (nothing added); legumes; plain potatoes and rice; fresh fruits; and fresh vegetables. All of these foods are healthy and delicious! The key is being careful to prepare these foods without other gluten-containing products and to eliminate the risk of contamination by any gluten-containing foods. Most dairy products can also be consumed as long as you are not lactose intolerant, which is quite common in people with celiac disease. There is large variety of gluten-free foods available, and that number will continue to grow as the number of people that are diagnosed with celiac disease increases.

FYI: If you suspect celiac disease in any way, it is of vital importance that you do not follow a gluten-free diet before having blood tests and/or a biopsy done. Following the diet before a proper diagnosis is made can interfere with test results and possibly produce an incorrect diagnosis. Don't assume because you are having problems becoming pregnant that eliminating gluten will do the trick. Speak with your healthcare provider first or you could be in for an even longer wait.

Celiac disease is not curable, and there are currently no drugs available to treat it. The only form of treatment is strict adherence to a 100-percent gluten-free diet for life. Not strictly adhering to a gluten-free diet can increase one's chance of developing other serious health problems down the line such as cancer in the intestinal wall as well as in other gastrointestinal areas. Some of the complications that accompany celiac disease can be healed or the risk lowered after adequate time on a gluten-free diet.

Celiac disease is a complex condition; this section has really only skimmed the surface. If this section has piqued your curiosity and you want to know more, check out *Tell Me What To Eat If I Have Celiac Disease* (Career Press) for more information on the disease and its treatment. The book contains a complete food list of what to eat and what not to eat, as well as recipes, resources, and more. If you have experienced infertility issues and suspect you have similar symptoms to the ones described here, speak with your healthcare provider about celiac disease. Sometimes you need to speak up and be your own advocate. If you have been diagnosed with celiac disease, be sure you are adhering faithfully to a gluten-free diet. Managing a gluten-free diet can be overwhelming at times, and if you are trying to conceive or have already become pregnant, it can be even more challenging. Working with a registered dietitian who specializes in celiac disease can help you to better understand and follow a gluten-free diet as well as address all of your individual nutritional challenges.

? Can my weight really make a difference?

The answer to that question is a definite yes. Studies have shown that body weight can most definitely affect fertility in both men and women. A healthy body weight is an important aspect of good health, and that includes reproductive health. Keep in mind we are discussing a *healthy* body weight and not an "ideal" body weight. A healthy weight is a weight that is best for you and not necessarily the lowest weight you think you can reach. As well, a healthy weight is not one single number but a range that is statistically related to good health. In other words, it is a weight that puts you at the lowest risk for health problems related to weight. The more overweight or underweight a woman is, the lower her chances are of becoming pregnant. It doesn't mean that becoming pregnant is impossible, but it does mean that it may be more difficult.

One way of determining a healthy weight is to calculate your BMI (Body Mass Index), which is a number based on body weight in relation to height. Women with a higher or lower BMI can have problems with *anovulation*, meaning they don't ovulate every cycle. However, it has been found that even women with regular cycles and no obvious fertility problems have a harder time conceiving if overweight. Reaching a healthy weight before trying to conceive will not only increase your chances of becoming pregnant but will also help to lower your risk of any possible complications once you become pregnant. Let's be realistic, though. It might not be possible for every woman to reach a healthy weight before trying to conceive. Don't let this discourage you if you fall into this category. Although pre-pregnancy weight within a normal BMI range is the healthiest goal, you might not have the luxury of time to gain or lose the weight to get to that point. Therefore, if your BMI is outside the normal range, consider delaying your date to start trying for just a short time so that you can at least begin taking the steps necessary to gradually improve your BMI by at least a few points. The postponement, as well as the time and effort you put into it, will be well worth it when you consider that it could make all the difference in your chances to conceive and possibly decrease your risk for miscarriage and health problems during pregnancy. If you are not at a healthy body weight and become pregnant, it is important that you work closely under the supervision of your healthcare provider and a registered dietitian to achieve the proper weight gain to sustain a healthy pregnancy. Chapter 2 will discuss more about BMI and the steps you need to take to achieve a healthier body weight.

? How old is too old to have a baby?

Is that biological clock ticking in your head? Are your family and friends reminding you of how quickly time is passing you by? It isn't unusual these days for women to start having children in their mid-30s or even well into their 40s. Times certainly have changed. In fact, about 20 percent of women in the United States have their first child after the age of 35. Although you may not feel your age and consider yourself in tip-top shape, when it comes to reproductive health, the medical community considers 35 years of age and older as *advanced maternal age*, or AMA. The major problem of delaying parenthood until after age 35 is that age has been found to decrease a woman's chances of becoming pregnant as well as increase the risk for miscarriage, pregnancy complications, and birth defects. Let's face it: our eggs have been with us since birth, so the older we get, the older and more fragile our eggs become, as well.

Potential problems with AMA include the decline of the ovaries to release eggs ready for fertilization, a decrease in the health and number of a woman's eggs, fluctuations in hormone levels, a higher risk of health problems that can interfere with fertility (such as endometriosis, blocked fallopian tubes, or fibroids), and an increased risk of miscarriage. Women over age 35 have a higher risk of developing high blood pressure and diabetes during pregnancy as well as experiencing stillbirth delivery, low birth weight babies, premature birth, and babies with birth defects. Women over age 35 are also more likely then younger women to have preexisting health conditions such as high blood pressure, diabetes, or heart problems, all of which can affect conception and/or pregnancy if not properly treated and controlled. And let's not leave men out of the picture. Older men can experience challenges, too, such as a decrease in sperm count.

That said, the good news is that it is not impossible for women in later life to become pregnant, experience a healthy pregnancy and deliver a healthy baby. If you do decide to delay having a child until later in life, you should visit your healthcare provider beforehand to discuss any potential risks as well as the steps you can take to minimize those risks and increase your chances of a successful pregnancy. This is especially important for a woman who has any type of preexisting chronic health problem(s) so that your healthcare provider can ensure your condition is being properly treated and can make any necessary changes in medications if needed. In addition, if you are over the age of 35 and have not conceived after 6 months of trying, you should again consult with your healthcare provider. Many fertility problems, even for women of AMA, can be treated successfully. Because women over the age of 35 have a higher risk of certain problems, they will experience more testing options that can help detect problems before, during, and after pregnancy. Whether a woman chooses to undergo testing is a personal decision and one she should make with the help of her healthcare provider. These tests might include ultrasounds, prenatal genetic testing, Quad Marker Screen, amniocentesis, and/or Chorionic Villus Sampling (CVS).

Good health prior to trying to conceive is essential for any woman, but even more so for women over the age of 35. General recommendations include:

- Consuming plenty of folic acid in your diet and through supplementation. Chapter 5 will provide you with more specific information on the recommendations for folic acid.

- Limiting your intake of caffeine. If you are a heavy coffee drinker or love your soft drinks, take a second look. You should limit your caffeine intake to no more then 200 milligrams (mg) per day. An 8-ounce cup of regular brewed coffee contains about 150 mg on average. A 12-ounce can of soda contains between 30 and

60 mg. Remember that other foods such as chocolate may also contain caffeine.

- Maintaining a healthy and well-balanced diet and eating a variety of foods each day to ensure you get all of the nutrients your body needs for good health and good reproductive health. Chapter 3 will provide you with more information on this topic.

- If you are not at a healthy weight, begin taking reasonable steps to reach a healthier BMI. Chapter 2 will provide you with more information.

- Being physically active most days of the week. If you are pregnant, speak with your healthcare provider about exercise that is safe.

- Quitting smoking if you're trying to conceive or pregnant. In fact, for good health, don't smoke at any time.

- Drinking alcohol in moderation or, if you're pregnant or suspect you're pregnant, stopping altogether.

Chapter 2

Weighing in on Your Fertility

It can be easy to take your fertility for granted. It is normal to believe that pregnancy will automatically happen when you are ready for it. But unfortunately for some, there can be many challenges (those we have control over and those that we don't) that can delay or halt the process. This chapter will discuss one challenge in particular, and that is the issue of body weight, something so many of us struggle with. If you want to successfully conceive, it is time to get in touch with your body and start to realize some of the steps you can take to make trying to conceive a more successful process.

A Healthy Weight for Trying to Conceive

Chapter 1 touched a bit on striving to reach a healthy weight. The reason for that is that, aside from the health risks it poses, an unhealthy weight (excess body fat or not enough body fat) can make it much harder to conceive. Whether you have a lot to lose or a little to lose, or even if your goal is to gain weight, weighing in before you begin your TTC journey will help you reach your ultimate goal much more quickly and with much less risk. Getting your weight as close to your healthy weight range as possible should definitely top your preconception to-do list. And the good news is that this is something you have more control over than you might think.

? How does weight affect my health and fertility?

Even though we touched on body weight briefly in Chapter 1, it is important enough to discuss it in more detail. There is no doubt that your body weight can have an impact on your chances of conceiving. Weighing either too much or too little can disrupt normal menstrual cycles and ovulation, making it difficult (or at times impossible) to become pregnant. Weighing in excess of your healthy range can not only lower your odds of becoming pregnant the natural way, but can also make it difficult if you are undergoing in-vitro fertilization or other assisted reproductive procedures. As we discussed earlier, not being within a healthy weight range can increase the risk for miscarriage and can put a pregnant woman at risk for developing problems such as high blood pressure (pre-eclampsia) and gestational diabetes (GDM), and increase the likelihood of a cesarean section. In fact, the risk of developing GDM during pregnancy is two-fold for overweight woman and that percentage risk increases as weight increases. Studies have also shown a strong correlation between obesity and insulin resistance, which can be another roadblock in the fertility process. Again, obesity is also a strong risk factor for PCOS, which can result in irregular menstrual cycles and ovulation problems, making it more difficult to become pregnant.

Let's not forget the effect obesity can have on your health, whether you are trying to conceive or not. Obesity is a major health issue in the United States and has increased significantly during the past two decades. In fact, almost two-thirds of the U.S. adult population is either overweight or obese. Both men and women who carry excess body weight are at greater risk for some of the following health problems:

- Hypertension (high blood pressure)
- Type 2 diabetes
- Osteoarthritis
- Dyslipidemia (such as high blood cholesterol and/or triglyceride levels)
- Stroke
- Coronary heart disease
- Sleep apnea
- Gallbladder disease
- Several types of cancer

The ultimate goal is to achieve and maintain a body weight that optimizes good overall health and good reproductive health. Eating healthily, staying physically active, and maintaining a healthy weight are all essential keys to a long and healthy life and successful conception. The choices you make every single day directly affect your health today, tomorrow, and in the future.

Not only can weight play a role in a woman's health before, during, and after pregnancy, but it can also extend to the health of her baby. Obesity can be an independent risk factor for birth defects (such as neural tube defects), fetal mortality, and pre-term delivery. This certainly doesn't mean you can't become pregnant or have a healthy baby if you weigh too much or too little for your body frame, but it does mean that it most likely will get in the way of getting pregnant successfully and can increase the risk of problems for the baby.

Not quite sure where your weight should be or how to get to that point in a fertility-friendly way? Read on for more information on healthy weight and how you can tip the scale in your favor. It is always important to talk with your healthcare provider concerning a practical goal that is right for you before starting to lose weight and/or beginning an exercise program.

FYI: Women who are suffering from or in the process of trying to recover from an eating disorder should refrain from the TTC process. Fertility can many times be compromised, sometimes severely, by an eating disorder, especially one that is currently untreated. If someone with an eating disorder is even able to become pregnant, the nutritional deprivation can put both the mother and baby at risk for complications. In addition, the psychological stress of gaining weight for the sake of the baby can make the situation even more dire. The good news is that taking the right steps to bring an eating disorder under control, with professional supervision, can help a woman increase her chances of becoming pregnant and carrying a healthy baby. If you suspect you have an eating disorder, speak with your healthcare provider before starting your TTC journey. Check out the Resources section for more information on eating disorders.

? How can I determine my healthy weight range?

We have talked a lot about BMI when it comes to determining a healthy weight. Sure, you can hop on the scale, but it won't provide all the information you need when it comes to your weight. BMI is one way to determine if extra pounds translate into a health risk. BMI is the measurement of weight relative to height and can determine whether you are at a healthy weight or if your weight is putting you at risk. Keep in mind that BMI is not a measurement of body fat so it can sometimes misclassify people. For example, someone with a lot of muscle mass may have a misleadingly high BMI, because BMI doesn't measure body fat and doesn't take into consideration that the majority of this person's body weight is coming from muscle and not fat. It can do the opposite for elderly people and underestimate BMI, not taking into account the muscle mass they have lost through the years. BMI can also misclassify women who are pregnant because it doesn't calculate the weight that is being carried in the form of fluids, additional blood, fat stores, and the baby. However, for the majority of us, BMI is a good indicator of what a healthy weight range should be.

You can crunch the numbers yourself by using this formula:

Weight in pounds [height in inches] squared × 703

Or use the chart on page 52 to easily find your BMI.

To use this BMI chart, locate your height in the left-hand column and follow the row across that height to find your weight. Follow that column of the weight up to the top to locate your BMI.

Now that you know your BMI, what exactly does it mean? Healthy weight is a range and not one single weight. The following will show you what range you fall into and what your BMI means for you:

BMI	Weight
Under 18.5	Underweight
18.5 to 24.9	Healthy Weight
25.0 to 29.9	Overweight
Over 30.0	Obese

Studies have concluded that for most woman, the most fertility-friendly range is somewhere in the healthy weight range. This is not a magic bullet, but it has shown to have numerous benefits. If you are not in that fertility-friendly range, don't despair! Keep reading for some tips on working toward this range to gain or lose the necessary weight. Every little bit counts, and small lifestyle and dietary changes are often all it takes to have the desired effect of improved fertility

? *Why does the shape of my body matter?*

BMI is only one factor in the attempt to assess weight. For an accurate assessment of weight related to health, it is also important to look at where you store fat. In typical healthcare fashion,

BMI	19	20	21	22	23	24	25	26	27	28	29	30	31	32	33	34	35
Height							Weight in Pounds										
4'10"	91	96	100	105	110	115	119	124	129	134	138	143	148	153	158	162	167
4'11"	94	99	104	109	114	119	124	128	133	138	143	148	153	158	163	168	173
5'	97	102	107	112	118	123	128	133	138	143	148	153	158	163	168	174	179
5'1"	100	106	111	116	122	127	132	137	143	148	153	158	164	169	174	180	185
5'2"	104	109	115	120	126	131	136	142	147	153	158	164	169	175	180	186	191
5'3"	107	113	118	124	130	135	141	146	152	158	163	169	175	180	186	191	197
5'4"	110	116	122	128	134	140	145	151	157	163	169	174	180	186	192	197	204
5'5"	114	120	126	132	138	144	150	156	162	168	174	180	186	192	198	204	210
5'6"	118	124	130	136	142	148	155	161	167	173	179	186	192	198	204	210	216
5'7"	121	127	134	140	146	153	159	166	172	178	185	191	198	204	211	217	223
5'8"	125	131	138	144	151	158	164	171	177	184	190	197	203	210	216	223	230
5'9"	128	135	142	149	155	162	169	176	182	189	196	203	209	216	223	230	236
5'10"	132	139	146	153	160	167	174	181	188	195	202	209	216	222	229	236	243
5'11"	136	143	150	157	165	172	179	186	193	200	208	215	222	229	236	243	250
6'	140	147	154	162	169	177	184	191	199	206	213	221	228	235	242	250	258
6'1"	144	151	159	166	174	182	189	197	204	212	219	227	235	242	250	257	265
6'2"	148	155	163	171	179	186	194	202	210	218	225	233	241	249	256	264	272
6'3"	152	160	168	176	184	192	200	208	216	224	232	240	248	256	264	272	279
6'4"	156	164	172	180	189	197	205	213	221	230	238	246	254	263	271	279	287
	Healthy Weight						Overweight					Obese					

the shape of our body, or where we store that excess fat, is compared to a fruit, either an apple or a pear.

- If you are shaped more like an apple, meaning you store and carry the majority of your fat in the stomach area and around your waist, you are at a higher risk for certain health problems such as cardiovascular disease, high blood pressure, type 2 diabetes, and certain types of cancer.

- If you are shaped more like a pear, meaning you store and carry the majority of your fat below the waist, in your hips, buttocks, and thighs, your shape does not put you at as much of a health risk as the "apples."

Most of us are painfully aware of where we store every little bit of fat, so you shouldn't have much problem figuring out which fruit you resemble. But if you just can't decide whether you look more like an apple or a pear, you can use your waist-to-hip ratio. Your waist-to-hip ratio can help determine, in a more scientific way, if the location of your body fat is putting you at greater risk for health problems related to your weight.

Follow these steps to figure out your waist-to-hip ratio:

1. Stand relaxed. Measure your waist at its smallest point (just above your hip bone) without sucking in your stomach or pulling the tape measure too tight.

2. Measure your hips by measuring the largest part of your buttocks and hips.

3. Divide your waist measurement by your hip measurement.

4. If this number is nearly or more than 1.0, you would be considered an apple shape.

5. If this number is considerably less than 1.0, you would be considered a pear shape.

Why is this important? We already know that women who weigh too much have a lower conception rate. However, it has been discovered that body fat distribution and where you carry most of your body fat may have an even greater impact. Researchers have found that overweight women with higher waist-to-hip ratios (the apple shapes) seem to have more difficulty getting pregnant than overweight women with lower waist-to-hip ratios (the pear shapes). So it seems that where you store fat on your body may be just as important, or maybe even more important, than how much excess body fat you have.

> *FYI: Your body shape, whether apple or pear, can be genetically determined. In other words, where you carry fat may have been passed down through your family tree. However, smoking and drinking too much alcohol can also contribute to excess fat in the stomach area. Genetic or not, if you don't have excess body fat to carry around you won't have to worry about where you carry it. Eating healthy and engaging in regular exercise can help you to lower excess body fat along with your risks for health problems not to mention increase your fertility health.*

? How does body fat affect my fertility hormones?

Both too much body fat and not enough body fat can affect fertility, and one of the reasons for this is the effect of weight on certain hormones. Body fat directly affects the release of estrogen, the hormone that stimulates the ovaries to produce and mature an egg, build up the uterine lining, and help regulate the menstrual cycle. Some of the estrogen our body uses is actually produced by our fat cells. If you are at a healthy weight and have a normal number of fat cells, you are most likely producing just the right amount of estrogen. If you have more fat cells then what is healthy for your body then you may be producing too much estrogen. If you are underweight, chances are you are not producing enough estrogen. Because it takes a delicate balance of hormones to regulate your menstrual cycle and keep the fertility cycle moving along, too much or too little estrogen can definitely cause the process to falter. In addition, excess body fat can cause increases in the hormone insulin along with increases in male sex hormones such as testosterone, which can hamper ovulation, making it harder and sometimes impossible to become pregnant. If you don't ovulate you can't get pregnant.

? Does his *weight matter?*

We don't want the men to feel left out when it comes to the numbers game. For his health and fertility's sake, it is just as important that he begins taking steps to reach a healthy weight if he has too high or too low of a BMI. Research has shown that overweight men are not as fertile as men who are at a healthy weight. Excess body weight in men tends to throw off hormone ratios by lowering testosterone levels and increasing estrogen levels, translating into a reduced production of the good swimming sperm.

Recent studies have also shown that too low of a BMI in men can significantly lower sperm count and concentration. Not as much is known about men being overweight or underweight where fertility is concerned compared to women, but suffice to say that men who are carrying too much weight or not enough weight can benefit from taking steps to reach a healthy weight, both from a fertility and an improved overall health standpoint.

Reaching a Healthy Weight

There are so many good reasons to reach a healthy weight, and if you are reading this book, trying to conceive successfully is probably at the top of your list. If you have a way to go to get to your healthy weight range, take heart in knowing that a little bit can go a long way. If you are on the overweight side of the coin, losing just 5 to 10 percent of your current weight can sometimes be just the ticket to improve ovulation and, therefore, your chances of becoming pregnant. If being underweight is your predicament, gaining just 5 to 10 pounds to start can sometimes be enough of a weight gain to restart and normalize ovulation and menstrual periods and improve your chances of becoming pregnant successfully. Don't stop there, though! Make sure that your long-term goal is to reach that weight range that will stamp you with a healthy BMI and lead you to better overall health.

The reality for someone who has been overweight or obese is that it is unlikely that he or she will reach a normal weight range prior to conception and/or pregnancy. If this is the case with you, nutritional counseling during pregnancy is highly recommended to ensure that a healthy pregnancy weight is reached and that healthy eating practices are put into place. This also goes for women who are underweight and who do not gain enough to reach a healthy weight prior to conceiving.

? How can I best lose weight?

The good news is that a modest weight loss will help to improve fertility for most women. If you are like most women, you want to lose weight in the quickest and easiest way possible. Who doesn't? But resist the urge to sign up for fad diets or any type of diet that promises quick weight loss. These types of diets usually involve deprivation of some kind, and that can easily deplete your body's stores of essential baby-making nutrients. Not to mention the fact that losing weight too quickly can mess with ovulation and/or menstrual cycles. Steer clear also of liquid diets, diet pills, or diet supplements that promise that tempting quick fix. Slow and steady wins the race to long lasting weight loss, better health, and improved fertility. Losing just 1 to 2 pounds per week is a safe and effective goal. The ultimate goal should not only be to increase fertility but to lose the weight and keep it off for good!

It doesn't take as much effort as you might think to begin losing or gaining weight. You can do it safely by adding or subtracting as little as 250 to 500 calories per day. For losing weight, that can be as simple as eliminating a regular can of soft drink and that midday candy bar. There is no need to drastically slash your food intake all at one time. Instead, try cutting back slowly. Making healthier choices by eliminating unhealthy foods and replacing them with healthier foods will most of the time automatically cut calorie intake. As your body becomes accustomed to this new calorie level, which you might notice by experiencing a weight plateau, it may be time to cut a bit more. The idea is that for a fertility friendly weight loss, you want to lose weight slowly, steadily, and in a healthy manner. Again, it doesn't take a whole lot to begin reversing the process and getting your cycles back on track.

> FYI: About 3,500 calories add up to one pound. Therefore, to lose one pound per week, you must split up a deficit of 3,500 calories over a week's time. Deducting 500 calories per day should result in a 1 pound per week weight loss.

The key is to worry less about every little calorie and concentrate more in general on eating nutrient-rich foods that make calories count, all while still keeping an eye on your portion sizes. This will ensure that you will be getting all the necessary nutrients your body needs, not only for good health, but also to support a healthy pregnancy. It is time to change bad habits into good ones, and that goes for eating as well as exercise. Here are just a few strategies that may help you begin losing weight in a way that is fertility friendly:

- Keep a daily food diary that includes what you eat, when you eat, and how much you eat. Write it down or find a free online food diary such as *www.fitday.com*. Review your diary frequently so that you can pinpoint and work on problem areas. Keeping a food diary can also help to keep you compliant and on track.

- Do *not* skip meals, and that includes breakfast. You won't save calories. Skipping a meal will lead to eating more than you should at the next meal and/or cause uncontrolled snacking throughout the day, both of which will pack on more calories than you need.

- Set realistic goals and don't expect to change all of your bad habits, or the habits that have caused that weight gain, all at one time. Work on changing habits one at a time. Once you have mastered one goal, move on to the next.

- Stick to a well-balanced and healthy eating routine. Healthier choices usually mean fewer calories, less fat, less sodium, and more nutritional value. The USDA's Dietary Guidelines for Americans can provide you with information on good dietary habits: *www.health.goc/ dietaryguidelines.*

- Cut back or cut out junk food such as sweets, soft drinks, fast food, and chips.

- Plan your healthy meals and snacks ahead of time so that you are always prepared.

- Become aware of and practice portion control.

- Avoid eating in front of the television (especially late night snacks) or computer or while doing other activities that keep you from paying attention to how much you are eating.

- Slow yourself down while eating. It takes a good 20 minutes for your brain to get the message you are full. Eating too quickly leads to eating too much.

- Use a smaller size plate for your food. It will help to keep your portions and calories under control and make you feel that you are getting a full plate of food.

- Plan and prepare more meals at home to keep from eating out too often. Restaurant meals tend to be high in calories, and it can sometimes be too tempting to make the right choices when eating out. Don't deprive yourself of eating out—make it an occasional outing instead of a regular habit—and work on making better choices when you do eat out.

- Learn how to read and use food labels to your advantage: *www.fda/Food/Labeling/Nutrition.*

- Check out the USDA's MyPlate Website to find a vast amount of information and hands-on tools that can help you lose weight sensibly and at the same time teach you what good nutrition really means: *www.choosemyplate.gov.*

- Incorporate physical activity most days of the week.

- If you feel you need more personal guidance, and many people do, turn to a registered dietitian who can educate, guide, motivate, and keep you on track to future success. You can check out *www.eatright.org* to find a dietitian in your area.

? How can I best gain weight?

If you have a BMI of less then 18.5, you are considered underweight, which could result in nutritional deficiencies in addition to fertility challenges. Putting on a few pounds should help increase your conception chances. However, this is not a green light to start scarfing down cookies, potato chips, candy, and other empty- calorie foods. As important as it is to lose weight in a healthy manner, it is just as important to gain weight in a healthy manner. Increasing exercise to build muscle, increasing calorie intake with healthy foods, and eating at least three full meals a day with healthy snacks in between can help you begin gaining weight. The solution is to eat extra calories from nutritious foods to ensure you get the proper nutrients that you need for good health and increased fertility, not to mention a healthy pregnancy.

Nutritious foods that can help tip the scale in your favor include healthy fats such as nuts, seeds, peanut butter, flaxseed oil, olive oil, or avocados; complex carbohydrates such as whole-grain pasta, brown rice, whole-grain breads and cereals, and beans; and dairy foods such as cheese, milk, yogurt, and ice cream (choose low-fat but not necessarily fat-free options when trying to gain weight). And don't forget your fruits and vegetables. Even though higher-fat foods can pack on calories, you still want to keep your overall eating plan moderate in total fat and concentrate on adding "good" fats as opposed to "bad" fats (saturated fats and trans fats). Here are a few tips to help get you started:

- If you have a small appetite and have a hard time getting all the food you need in a day, try spreading out your food intake and eating five to six meals and/or snacks per day.

- Drink fluids before and after meals instead of with meals so that you leave more room for food calories.

> FYI: There are just as many miracle weight gain products and supplements out there as there are weight loss products. Whether you are trying to gain or lose weight the same advice applies: if it sounds too good to be true it probably won't work. Don't waste your money on expensive supplements; spend it on good nutritious foods instead. If needed, there are some reliable calorie boosting supplements on the market, but you should speak with your healthcare provider and/or dietitian before using one.

- Try a few calorie-adding tricks such as topping your usual foods with grated cheese; preparing hot oatmeal with milk instead of water; adding seeds, nuts, olives, and/or avocados to salads; adding a few tablespoons of dry milk powder to soups, casseroles, or mashed potatoes; and spreading peanut butter on your breakfast toast.

- Choose healthier beverages such as juice, milk, smoothies, or milkshakes instead of diet or regular soft drinks that add no nutritional value.

- Exercise is great for good health and weight loss and yes, even if you are trying to gain weight it can have its perks. Exercise can build muscle, which can put bulk on your frame and pounds on the scale. It can also help to increase your appetite. However, if you are trying to gain weight and not seeing results and you vigorously work out often, you may be burning too many calories for what you are trying to eat. At this point you may want to look at toning your exercise down a notch or two. And just like those trying to lose weight, slow and steady should be your motto. If you are having problems gaining weight and/or maintaining your weight, seek help from your healthcare provider to rule out any health problems.

? How much weight do I need to gain once I become pregnant?

Once you become pregnant you will eventually begin to gain weight. However, there are recommendations as to how much this should be, depending on your weight and BMI as you enter pregnancy. Those women who gain more weight than needed during pregnancy are more at risk to become overweight after pregnancy and throughout their lifetime, compared to women who gain a healthy amount of weight during pregnancy. Recommendations as to how much weight a woman should gain during pregnancy is dependent on her BMI before becoming pregnant.

Pre-pregnancy BMI	BMI	Total Weight Gain Range (lbs)
Underweight	<18.5	28–40
Normal weight	18.5–24.9	25–35
Overweight	25.0–29.9	15–25
Obese (includes all classes)	≥30.0	11–20

Source: Institute of Medicine, May 2009

Although this chart gives you an idea of the amount of total weight gain recommended for pregnant women, it is always important to speak with your healthcare provider concerning the amount of weight gain that is right for *you*.

> FYI: According to the American Pregnancy Association, even though weight gain during pregnancy depends on a number of factors such as height, body type, and pre-pregnancy weight, most women carrying twins are encouraged to gain between 35 and 45 pounds. Women who are carrying triplets are encouraged to gain between 50 and 60 pounds.

Exercise and Its Many Benefits

It is pretty hard to deny the importance of regular exercise. Not only is it essential for good health, weight management, and a long life, but it may be another piece of the puzzle when it comes to trying to conceive. You don't necessarily have to be fit to get pregnant but there is a very good chance it could help. You don't have to be a star athlete or spend hours at the gym. The key is to exercise moderately and regularly. Researchers believe that a moderate exercise program that promotes overall fitness (about 30 minutes a day) can help boost fertility, not to mention health, for most people. If you are trying to lose weight, however, that time frame may need to be increased. Even if you cannot do all of your exercise at once, you can break it up during the day. Experts say three or more 10-minute sessions can be just as good as doing it all at once.

Exercise can help you to lose a few pounds, maintain a healthy weight, relieve stress, boost mood, increase self-esteem, improve sleep, and decrease your risk for a number of health issues, all of which can make your baby-making efforts more productive. In addition, exercise helps keep insulin and blood sugar in check, both of which are important for fertility. On the flip side, excessive exercise (such as marathon running or competitive athletics) can halt ovulation or cause erratic ovulation for some women. If you already exercise on a regular basis, pat yourself on the back and take heart. Your good exercise habits will carry you through the stage of trying to conceive and pregnancy as well as later stages of your life including middle age, menopause, and beyond. Keep it a lifelong habit! Your body and your health will thank you. Always talk to your healthcare provider about your workout routine before trying to conceive and especially if you become pregnant.

FYI: Drinking plenty of water before, during, and after exercise will help you and your muscles stay well-hydrated.

? What is the best kind of exercise?

The best fertility-friendly exercise should not differ all that much from that of someone exercising for good health. Your routine should be moderate, but what is moderate for you will depend on your current fitness level, so adjust accordingly. For someone who runs consistently, a 3-mile run may be a walk in the park, but for someone just getting started, this would be way over the top. Some good exercises to consider if you are just getting started include walking, swimming, dancing, Pilates, yoga, mild cardio workout, light weight training, stationary biking, and other low-impact workouts. Sticking to lower impact means you can most likely continue with your routine once you become pregnant (with your doctor's permission, of course). However, for women who are already physically fit, some vigorous activity may be okay. Again, it is always best to speak with your healthcare provider.

No matter what you decide to do, a well-balanced exercise routine should include a combination of aerobic exercise, resistance or strength training, warm-up/stretching/balance activities, and plenty of activities of daily living.

- Aerobic Exercise: The word *aerobic* literally means "with air." Therefore in aerobic exercise your muscles require an increased supply of oxygen. Aerobic activity is also known as cardio activity because it also speeds your heart rate and improves your lung and heart fitness. Examples of these activities include brisk walking, jogging, swimming, jumping rope, biking, and stair-climbing.

- Resistance/Strength Training: This type of activity helps to build and maintain muscles and bones by working them against gravity. Strength training is used for improving muscle strength and tone. In men, it will increase muscle size, and for women, it usually means more tone without significant muscle size increase. This can include using free weights such as dumbbells and/or weight machines, or stretch bands for resistance training.

- Warm-up/Stretching/Balance Activities: These types of activities can help to improve physical stability and flexibility, which can help reduce the risk for injuries and help you to move around more easily. The best time to stretch is when your muscles are already warmed up to prevent injury. Try to hold each stretch for at least 15 seconds and *never* bounce. Stretch to the point of mild tension but not pain.

Exercise is not the only way to burn calories. In addition to exercise, it is essential to keep yourself moving throughout the day; in other words, increase your activities of daily living. Don't get me wrong—exercise is great, but if you really want to burn more calories, think of adding the following activities to your exercise routine each and every day. The more you move your body, the better!

- Take the stairs instead of the elevator.
- Park at the far end of the parking lot for a longer walk, if it is safe.
- Forget the drive-thru at the bank; park and walk in.
- If you have a sit-down job, get up every 30 minutes or so and move around.
- Play actively with your kids instead of watching from the sidelines.
- Take the dog for regular walks.
- Wash your car yourself instead of taking it to the car wash.
- While on the phone, walk around the house instead of sitting on the couch.

The most important factor about exercise and staying active is to find something that you enjoy so that you are apt to stick with it and perform it on a regular basis. If you are currently a couch potato or an occasional exerciser at most, start slowly and work your way up. If you are really not sure where to start, walking is always a good choice. You can also look into speaking with a personal trainer at your local gym or recreation center.

? What about his exercise routine?

Men need to take a look at their workout routine or the sports they are playing, as well, if they are trying to conceive with their partner. With any kind of rough sports, protective gear should be worn. That might go without saying, but during the TTC process it is even more important. Some experts believe that too much cycling for men, more than about 12 hours a week, may have an adverse effect on fertility. Although exercise can help boost fertility, it is still not a good idea to overdo it if you want to be at your baby-making peak. Intense workouts can change hormone levels and may even lower sperm count. As for post-workout relaxation, steer clear of hot tubs, saunas, or steam rooms that overheat you, all of which can impair sperm production. Men who don't work out at all should think about getting in the game because they will be more likely to encounter fertility challenges if they don't.

? How do I know if I am working out too hard or not hard enough?

It is vital to an effective workout program to be sure you are working hard enough but not too hard. Another word for this is *intensity*, or how hard your body is working during aerobic activity. You can test yourself in a few ways. One quick way is the "talk test." If you can comfortably carry on a conversation while exercising you are working out at a moderate intensity and are doing fine. At this point you have raised your heart rate enough to break a sweat. The next step is a vigorous activity level, where your heart rate goes up even more and you are breathing hard and fast, making it hard to hold a conversation. A mix of the two is a good combination, once you get to that level. Start at a lower intensity level and work your way up to a more vigorous one over time. If you get to the point that you can barely catch your breath and cannot carry on a conversation, you need to slow yourself down a bit. On the other hand, if you can babble along without barely taking a breath in between sentences, you need to step it up. You should feel like you are working yourself but not to the point of pure exhaustion.

FYI: Be careful not to get overheated. This isn't harmful to your fertility but it can be harmful if you are pregnant but don't know it. Go ahead and work up a sweat—just be cautious of extremely hot environments such as running outside on a really hot day.

There is a mathematical way to calculate your target heart rate, or the number of times your heart beats per minute. This will let you know if you are working out in your training or target heart rate zone. In general, the target rate for women is somewhere between 50 and 85 percent of their maximum heart rate. This is only an estimate, but will let you know whether you are working out too hard or not hard enough.

To calculate your target heart rate:

1. Calculate your estimated maximum heart rate:
    220 – your age

2. Calculate your lower range:
    Maximum heart rate × .50 (50%)

3. Calculate your upper range:
    Maximum heart rate × .85 (85%)

Example: 30-year-old woman

1. 220 – 30 = 190 maximum heart rate

2. 190 × .50 = 95 lower range

3. 190 × .85 = 162 upper range

FYI: Some experts such as the American College of Obstetricians and Gynecologists (ACOG) recommend that during pregnancy, women should exercise at least 30 minutes per day without any specific heart rate limits. Other experts recommend keeping your heart rate under 140 beats per minute, especially in the first trimester. Every woman is different, so once you become pregnant check with your healthcare provider concerning the safest exercise routine for you.

This means that her target zone is between 95 and 162 beats per minute. So if it falls below 95, she needs to step it up, and if it goes higher then 162, she needs to ease up. If you are new to exercising you should aim for the lower range of your target rate. As you become more physically fit, you can gradually build up to the higher end.

To keep yourself in your target zone, you need to check your heart rate throughout your exercise session. To find your pulse, place your index and middle fingers over the outside of your opposite wrist and press lightly. Once you have located your pulse, use the second hand of a watch or clock and count the beats you feel in a 15-second span. Multiply that number by four. The result is your heart rate.

Chapter 3

Diet Rules to Eat By

As you try to conceive and prior to becoming pregnant, your health can have a huge impact on your probability of success. In addition to getting your weight in order, there is your diet to think about. What are you eating? Are you eating right? What *should* you be eating? Now that you have decided it is time to bring a new life into the world, you need to take a hard look at what you eat each day. Is it hurting your chances or helping your chances of conception? It is time to find out.

Because the cornerstone of a fertility-friendly diet is adopting a generally healthier eating style and lifestyle in general, this chapter will discuss how everyone can begin to do just that. It will also point out a few specifics about eating in a particularly fertility-friendly way.

The Importance of Eating a Fertility-Friendly Diet

Most of us realize that a healthy diet is essential for good health; we have come to realize it is just as important for successful conception. Eating a healthy diet and picking out some powerhouse foods that might benefit fertility even more won't guarantee a pregnancy; however, new research is finding promising evidence that good nutrition can have a positive impact on fertility. And let's not forget that eating healthily is easy to try, is an option available to everyone, and will set the stage for a healthy pregnancy and beyond. The sooner you begin a healthier way of eating, the better, and starting before you even begin trying to conceive puts you ahead of the game. Not sure exactly how to start when it comes to eating a fertility-friendly, healthy diet? Read on!

Exploring the USDA MyPlate

We make numerous food choices each and every day. Whether these choices seem trivial or significant, made over and over through time, they can have a major impact on our overall health, our weight, and our reproductive health. Eating a healthy and well-balanced diet and engaging in regular physical activity are two of the best personal investments anyone can make. There is no secret to a healthy diet and a healthy lifestyle; there's just solid advice. Lucky for us, the USDA (United States Department of Agriculture) gives us just that in the MyPlate Icon. MyPlate is an online concept that offers dietary recommendations, nutrition education, up-to-date information, personalized eating plans, and interactive tools to help you plan and asses your food choices based on the Dietary Guidelines for Americans, which we will discuss next. I'll bet you didn't even realize you have all of this right at your fingertips!

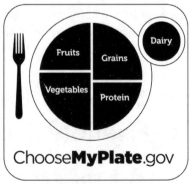

Source: U.S. Department of Agriculture
www.usda.gov, www.choosemyplate.gov

The MyPlate icon was designed to remind all Americans in a very simple way to eat healthfully. MyPlate illustrates the five food groups using a familiar mealtime visual that we all use, a plate and a place setting. MyPlate includes fruits, vegetables, grains, and proteins on the plate with a serving of dairy off to the side. You can check out the full-color image by visiting the Website. Individual foods and/or numbers of servings are not shown specifically in the icon; instead, the graphic leads us to seek more information by visiting *www.choosemyplate.gov* for a one-stop-shopping–type deal, and it is all completely free! This is the perfect place to go to put together a plan that will help balance your intake of the food groups, find menus and recipes, determine serving sizes, point out which foods are healthier to eat, estimate your daily caloric needs, and provide you with all of the general information you need to eat more healthily and maintain or reach a healthy weight.

MyPlate allows you to take action on the Dietary Guidelines by making changes in three areas:

Balancing Calories

- Enjoy your food, but eat less.
- Avoid oversized portions.

Foods to Increase

- Make half your plate fruits and vegetables.
- Make at least half your grains whole grains.
- Switch to fat-free or low-fat (1%) milk.

Foods to Reduce

- Compare sodium in foods like soup, bread, and frozen meals, and choose the foods with the lower numbers.
- Drink water instead of sugary drinks.

ChooseMyPlate has loads of interactive tools that can help you personalize a healthy diet plan that is just right for you.

- **Daily Food Plan:** This tool will estimate your calorie level along with a food plan. You can print out a mini-poster of your food plan along with a worksheet to help you track your progress. Tailored Daily Food Plans are also available for preschoolers (2–5 years) and women who are pregnant or breastfeeding.

- **Food Groups:** This section provides you with in-depth information about each food group, including suggested serving sizes, how much you need, and how to choose the best foods in that group.

- **Food Tracker:** This section will provide you with a detailed analysis of your current eating and exercise habits.

- **Food Menu Planner:** Here you can determine your nutritional goals as well as plan food choices and menus to meet those goals.

- **My Food-A-Pedia:** This section provides quick access to food information. Find out what food group any food belongs to and its calorie content per serving. You can also use this tool to compare two foods.

FYI: The Dietary Guidelines for Americans and MyPlate are not meant for people with specific health conditions. People with chronic health conditions should consult with their healthcare provider and a registered dietitian to determine a dietary intake that is appropriate for them.

Discovering the Dietary Guidelines for Americans

The Dietary Guidelines for Americans are issued and updated jointly by the Department of Health and Human Services (HHS) and the Department of Agriculture (USDA) every five years. They are the foundation of MyPlate and together they work hand-in-hand. The 2010 Dietary Guidelines for Americans, along with MyPlate, provide scientifically-based advice for people 2 years and older and focus on preventing and reducing overweight and obesity through better eating and exercise habits. The Guidelines emphasize a total diet approach by urging Americans to reduce calories by watching portion sizes; making more nutrient-rich food choices such as fruits, veggies, whole grains, and low-fat and fat-free milk and milk products; eating fewer calories from foods such as solid fats and added sugars; and by moving more.

All Americans are urged to read the Dietary Guidelines for Americans to become educated about what is recommended for a healthy diet and beneficial physical activity. Eating healthily and being physically active should not be just a "diet" or something you do temporarily to become pregnant and/or lose weight; rather, it should become something you do for the rest of your life. That is the key to adopting healthier lifestyle habits that will help to reduce your risk for numerous chronic diseases and increase your chances for a longer life. Each Guideline consists of key recommendations, with some targeting specific populations, including women who are trying to become pregnant or who are already pregnant.

Some of the more specific recommendations:

- Balancing calories to manage weight, including maintaining appropriate calorie balance during each stage of life: childhood, adolescence, adulthood, pregnancy and breastfeeding, and old age.

- Increasing physical activity
- Foods and food components to reduce, such as sodium, saturated fats, dietary cholesterol, trans fats, solid fats, added sugars, refined grains, and alcohol.
- Foods and nutrients to increase, such as a variety of fruits and vegetables; whole grains; low-fat or fat-free milk and milk products; a variety of leaner protein sources (seafood, lean meats and poultry, eggs, beans, peas, soy products, nuts and seeds); oils to replace solid fats; and foods higher in potassium, dietary fiber, calcium, and vitamin D.
- Women capable of becoming pregnant should choose foods that supply heme iron, a form of iron that is more readily absorbed by the body, additional iron sources, and enhancers of iron absorption including foods rich in vitamin C.
- Women capable of becoming pregnant should consume 400 mcg per day of synthetic folic acid (from fortified foods and/or supplements) in addition to foods rich in folate from a varied diet.
- Building healthy eating patterns that meet your nutrient needs through time at an appropriate calorie level, accounting for all foods and beverages and assessing how well they fit within your healthy eating pattern, and always following food safety recommendations when preparing and eating foods to help reduce the risk for foodborne illnesses.

To find out the details of these recommendations and more, check out: *www.cnpp.usda.gov/dietaryguidelines.htm.*

Focusing on Fats

Even with all the bad press fat gets, it is important to realize that some dietary fat is essential to our survival. We need moderate amounts to perform important functions such as carrying, absorbing, and storing fat-soluble vitamins (A, D, E, and K). Dietary fat is used as an energy source and is stored in our fat cells for future energy needs.

Keep in mind that a little fat goes a long way—hence the recommendations from MyPlate and the Dietary Guidelines for Americans that tell us to go easy on the fats. Your goal should not be to eliminate all the fat from your diet but to limit total fat and consume most of your fat intake from healthier fat sources. In fact, reducing your total fat intake too much can lead to fertility problems. Although "good" fats are actually essential to a healthy diet, fat is still loaded with calories; so, eat them sparingly but *do* include them. The Dietary Guidelines for Americans follows the Institute of Medicine (IOM) and recommends consuming no more then 20 to 35 percent of your total daily caloric intake from fat, with the majority coming from healthy fats and as little as possible coming from the saturated and trans fats. Eating too much of any fat can cause weight gain because of its high caloric content. Eating too much saturated fat and trans fat not only can cause weight gain but can put you at risk for serious health problems such as heart disease, stroke, and certain types of cancer.

Most of the fats that you eat should be made up of "good" fats, including polyunsaturated fats (PUFA), omega-3 fatty acids, and monounsaturated fats (MUFA), and less of the "bad" fats, including saturated fats and trans fats. The more foods you eat that contain "bad" fats, the less room there is for healthier foods, which all translates into decreased fertility. On the flip side, eating fewer "bad" fats while adding in moderate amounts of the "good" fats may just give your fertility a boost.

When we talk about "good" fats we are talking about the unsaturated sources that, as mentioned previously, include monounsaturated fats, polyunsaturated fats, and omega-3 fatty acids. "Good" fats are heart healthy and have health-promoting effects. In fact, research shows that omega-3 fatty acids, a type of polyunsaturated fat, can help reduce inflammation and may have the power to reduce the risk for heart disease, cancer, arthritis, and a host of other health issues. They may help lower total cholesterol, increase HDL (good) cholesterol, lower triglycerides, lower blood pressure, possibly help alleviate some of the symptoms of depression as well as other psychological disorders, improve skin disorders, and the list goes on as more research is completed. In addition, omega-3 fats, especially DHA, are essential to the brain and eye development of a growing fetus. In fish, these fats are found in the form of EPA (eicosapentaenoic acid) and DHA (docoshexaeonic acid), which are two potent forms of omega-3 fats that provide the greatest health benefits. Omega-3 fats are also found in plant sources in the form of ALA (alpha linolenic acid), but it is the preformed DHA in seafood that the body most prefers. The March of Dimes recommends that pregnant women get at least 200 mg of DHA every day.

Depending on a woman's fertility problems, some studies suggest that a diet full of omega-3 fatty acids may increase a woman's chances of becoming pregnant. However, don't go overboard with it! Too much omega-3, especially in the form of supplements such as fish oil capsules, can have negative health implications for some people. If you plan to increase your intake, speak with your healthcare provider first and try to get most of your intake from food sources.

Not sure where to find these fabulous fats? Here is a list of some sources of each. This is not a complete list but it will give you a good place to start.

Sources of monounsaturated fats:

- Olive oil and olives
- Canola and peanut oil
- Sunflower and sesame oil
- Avocados
- Nuts, including hazelnuts, macadamia nuts, almonds, Brazil nuts, cashews, and pecans
- Seeds, including sesame seeds, pumpkin seeds, and sunflower seeds
- Peanut butter

Sources of polyunsaturated fats:

- Vegetable oils such as soybean, corn, and safflower oil
- Nuts, including walnuts, pine nuts, and butternuts
- Fatty fish and seafood (in the form of omega-3 fatty acids)

Sources of omega-3 fats:

- Coldwater fish such as salmon, halibut, mackerel, herring, anchovies, tuna, and sardines (see Chapter 4 for guidelines on eating fish and more information on omega-3 fats).
- Flaxseeds, ground or whole, and flaxseed oil (it is not recommended to use flaxseed oil supplements during pregnancy)
- Walnuts
- Soybeans
- Omega-3 fortified foods such as milk, eggs, peanut butter, and margarine

When we talk about "bad" fats we are talking about saturated fat sources as well as trans fats. These types of fat do nothing good for you. Too much of either of these fats will wreak havoc on your health and put you at higher risk for heart disease, stroke, and cancer, as well as possibly slowing down your efforts to get pregnant. Recent research has found that consuming too many trans fats specifically may have a direct correlation to a decline in fertility.

Saturated fats can be found naturally in most animal-based foods, such as whole or low-fat dairy products, meat, poultry, and butter. In addition you can find it in many baked goods and fried foods, especially fast foods. Even though most vegetable oils contain more unsaturated fats there are a few that contain more saturated fats, including coconut oil, palm oil, and palm kernel oil. Trans fats, which you should eat as little of as possible, are found naturally in a few foods such as full-fat dairy products and fatty meats. They are also created when a liquid vegetable oil is made more solid by the addition of hydrogen, a process called *hydrogenation*. These more solid fats gained popularity with manufacturers because they increase the shelf-life and improve the flavor of many baked and processed foods. Trans fats are most commonly found in fast foods, some processed snack foods and baked goods, stick margarines, and shortening. If you are a label reader, keep in mind that even though a food label states "trans-fat free," it can still contain up to 0.5 gram/serving of food. Eat enough of that food and it surely is not free of trans fats. It may not sound like much, but when experts recommend eating no more then one percent of your total daily calories in this form, which would calculate to 2 grams per day on a typical 2,000-calorie diet, that little 0.5 gram seems like a lot more! If you really want to ensure your food doesn't contain any trans fats, check the ingredient label and make sure it does not list partially hydrogenated oil.

You can lower your consumption of "bad" fats and increase your consumption of "good" fats by following a few simple strategies:

- Include leaner cuts of meat and eat poultry without skin.
- Prepare a vegetarian dish with legumes, nuts, or seeds once or twice a week.
- Include fish as part of your weekly meal plan.
- Limit your intake of baked goods, cookies, and other processed snack foods and instead grab a piece of fruit or a handful of nuts or seeds. Keep healthier snacks on hand and unhealthy foods out of the house so you are not tempted.
- Forget mayo on your sandwich and drizzle a little olive oil or smash up avocados for a yummy spread.
- Use olive oil in place of butter or margarine when possible, such as on streamed vegetables or on garlic bread.
- Flavor foods with herbs and spices instead of butter or margarine.
- Create your own salad dressings instead of using commercial dressings, which are often overly processed and

full of saturated fats. Mix olive oil with a little lemon juice and your favorite herbs and spices for a quick and healthy dressing.

- Add some chopped avocado, along with seeds or nuts, as a healthy salad topping.

- Use ground flaxseed in your favorite yogurt or smoothie.

Carbohydrates Count

Carbohydrates have received a bad rap the last few years. Confusion surrounds the theories of low carbs or no carbs. This important nutrient is blamed for the obesity problem, for diabetes, and the list goes on. The fact is that carbohydrates alone do not make you fat, nor do they cause diabetes as some fad diets out there might have you believe. Eating too much food in general, regardless of which foods you get your energy from, and not burning enough calories is what leads to unwanted weight gain. In fact, the right carbs, in moderation, are an essential part of a well-balanced diet, whether you are trying to lose weight, stabilize your blood sugar, or become pregnant. They key is balancing your intake of carbs, fats, and protein appropriately and choosing the healthiest foods to provide these important nutrients.

Carbs beat out both fats and proteins when it comes to how readily they are converted into glucose (sugar that circulates in your bloodstream), which makes them an ideal source of energy for the body. When we talk about carbohydrates we are including starch and sugar as well as fiber. But it is starch and sugar that contribute to our energy needs, and the one you choose more often can make all the difference.

Carbohydrates are classified in two categories: simple (sugars) and complex (starches). Even though there are two different types of carbohydrates, they are both eventually broken down into glucose, which is then converted into energy for the body to use. Simple carbohydrates are sugars or carbohydrates in their simplest form. Simple carbs or sugars come from or are added to foods and beverages such as honey, jelly, candy, table sugar, cookies, cakes, ice cream, soft drinks, fruit drinks, and other sweet treats and beverages. Simple carbs are sometimes referred to as "empty calories" because they provide calories but not much in the way of nutritional value. In most cases, the simpler a carb is, the faster it is broken down into glucose, which is then released into your bloodstream. This can sometimes wreak havoc on your blood sugar levels, causing peaks and drops. Not all simple sugars are bad, though. These sugars can also occur naturally in foods such as fructose (found in fruit) or lactose (found in dairy products), which are hardly classified as empty calories! When three or more sugar units are linked together they become complex carbohydrates, more commonly known as starches. These types of carbs are found in foods such as grains, pasta, rice, vegetables, potatoes, fruits, breads, legumes, nuts, and seeds. Unlike simple carbs, complex carbs take a little while longer to break down, therefore allowing for a slower release of glucose along with more stable blood sugar levels. In addition to being found circulating in the blood as glucose, carbohydrates are stored in the muscle and liver as glycogen for future energy stores. Your carbohydrate stores influence how long you can exercise and still feel good. When your muscle and liver glycogen stores get too low you may, "hit the wall" and feel fatigued during exercise. If you eat more carbohydrates than you need and burn, the excess is stored as body fat. Adults should get 45 to 65 percent of their total calories from carbohydrates, with the bulk coming from complex carbs versus simple carbs, especially the empty-calorie ones. The exception here is fruit and dairy foods. Even though they contain simple sugars they are also chock full of healthy nutrients, with fruit containing fiber, as well. Not only should you shoot for a greater number of complex carbs, but choosing whole grains will contribute even more in the way of fiber and nutrients.

Go for the Whole Grains

Now that we know a little bit about what carbs are and how much of them we need for a well-balanced diet and good reproductive health, let's get more specific about some of the healthy foods that make up the carbohydrate group. Grains are an important source of complex carbohydrates. They include foods made from wheat, rice, oats, cornmeal, barley, and other cereal grains. They are found in a lot of your favorite foods such as breads, pasta, rice, cereals, crackers, tortillas, popcorn—and the list goes on. It is never as simple as it looks, though. Grains are broken down into two groups: whole grains and refined grains. And one of these groups is much better for your health and fertility than the other.

Whole grains are more then just grains. They are nutritional powerhouses that also contribute fiber as well as additional essential nutrients. Whole grains are termed "whole" because they contain the entire grain kernel (bran, endosperm, and germ). All three of these layers are vital because they supply nutrients such as antioxidants, B vitamins, vitamin E, iron, healthy fats, protein, complex carbohydrates, and fiber. While a whole grain contains all parts of the grain kernel, a refined grain contains only the very inner portion of the endosperm. Therefore refined grains are missing all the nutrients the other two layers provide. Refined grains start out as whole grains but are processed and milled to have the bran and germ layers removed. This provides a product that is finer in texture and has a longer shelf-life. However, this isn't much of a trade-off because the process strips away fiber, iron, and essential vitamins such as B vitamins. Refined grains are found in foods such as white bread, white flour, baked goods, flour tortillas, white rice, and white pasta. In an effort to make refined grains more nutritious, many of them are "enriched," meaning certain nutrients, such as iron and B vitamins, are added back after the milling process. However, certain nutrients, including some kinds of fiber, cannot be added back, so they still don't stack up to whole grains. That pretty much gives you an answer as to which type of grain is best for good health.

Research has shown that eating too many refined grains along with simple carbohydrates can, in some women, upset the finely tuned balance of reproductive hormones, resulting in changes that can throw off ovulation and therefore lessen their chances for becoming pregnant. Your goal should be not only to choose complex carbs more often but also to go one step further and choose whole grains more often then refined grains. In a nutshell, it isn't so much the amount of carbohydrates you eat (though you should moderate them for a well-balanced diet) but the quality and type of carbohydrates that you eat more often that may increase or decrease your fertility.

The Dietary Guidelines for Americans recommend that adults eat at least half of their grains as whole grains, which adds up to about three to five servings of whole grains daily. Serving sizes of a few foods in the grain group include 1 slice of bread, 1/2 English muffin,1/2 cup cooked cereal, 3 cups popcorn, 1/2 cup cooked rice, 1/2 cup cooked pasta, and one 6-inch tortilla.

If you are not exactly sure which foods are whole grains, here is a list to help you get started:

- Barley
- Buckwheat
- Bulgur
- Corn
- Oats, including oatmeal
- Popcorn
- Quinoa
- Rice, wild and brown
- Rye, whole
- Whole-grain couscous
- Whole-wheat or whole-grain breads
- Whole-wheat flour
- Whole-wheat pasta

FYI: When choosing whole-grain products, read labels carefully. Just because bread is brown and/or states "wheat" on the label does not mean it is made from whole-wheat flour and is therefore a whole grain. Even words such as "multi-grain," "stone-ground," "cracked wheat," "100-percent wheat," "bran," or "seven grain" do not guarantee that a food contains whole grains. Look for the word "whole" on the food, for example "whole-wheat" or "whole grain," and check to see if whole grains appear near or at the top of the ingredients list to ensure you are buying a whole-grain product.

Don't Forget Your Fruits and Vegetables

There was a reason Mom always reminded you to eat your fruits and vegetables! These foods are the most natural foods we have and are another way to make sure you get your fill of complex carbs as well as all of the essential nutrients for good health. It's impossible to deny the fact that fruits and vegetables are good for you. These foods provide an abundance of vitamins, minerals, fiber, antioxidants, and phytonutrients, all of which contribute to better health and include all the nutrients that are so vital for good reproductive health. Eating more fruits and vegetables can reduce the risk for stroke, heart disease, type 2 diabetes, and even some types of cancers. Just making the simple change of eating fruit in place of sweets, junk foods, or other foods with added sugar and fat, and adding more vegetables at dinner may help you lose weight, maintain a healthy weight more easily, and increase your chances of conception. Next time you need a good crunch or that sweet tooth is nagging at you, pick up a sweet piece of fruit or a crunchy vegetable for a nutritional boost. In fact, the best way to make sure you eat these foods is to make sure you have them in the house. Your health and your fertility will thank you for it!

When it comes to fruit, you can enjoy it fresh, frozen, canned, or dried. Any or all will do the trick. If choosing canned fruit, pick one packed in its own juice as opposed to syrup. Fruit is an excellent source of vitamins A and C as well as potassium and is a boundless source of disease-fighting phytonutrients. In its whole form it is a great source of fiber, too! The more variety of fruit you eat, the more of a nutritional punch it will make in your daily intake. One serving of fruit equals 1 cup of fruit or 100-percent fruit juice, or 1/2 cup dried fruit. Most adults should shoot for at least 2 cups of fruit daily.

Vegetables can be enjoyed many ways, including raw, cooked, fresh, frozen, canned, or dried. They provide loads of vitamins, minerals, antioxidants, phytonutrients, and fiber, and as an added bonus, they are very low in calories. If choosing canned, go for the "no sodium added" versions or rinse them before preparing to minimize the amount of sodium that canned foods contain. Choose a variety of veggies and colors from all five vegetable subgroups (dark green, orange, legumes or dried beans, starchy vegetables, and other vegetables) for the most beneficial nutritional intake. The deeper the color of a vegetable, the more nutrition it is providing you. One serving of vegetables equals 1 cup of raw or cooked vegetables or vegetable juice, or 2 cups raw leafy greens. Most adults should shoot for at least 2.5 to 3 cups of vegetables daily.

FYI: For more fiber, you should choose whole fruit as opposed to fruit juice. However, when buying fruit juice pay close attention to the wording. Stay away from "fruit drinks" or "fruit cocktails" because they generally contain quite a bit of added sugar and very little actual fruit juice. Instead choose juice products that state "100-percent fruit juice."

A Little on Fiber

Fiber is a type of complex carbohydrate that is found only in plants and is frequently referred to as "roughage." Unlike other carbohydrates, the body does not digest or absorb fiber completely, so it doesn't contribute many calories the way other carbs do. Because of this, fiber is not considered a nutrient; however, you can still find it listed on food nutrient labels to help you choose fiber-rich foods. Fiber essentially travels in and back out of the body, but don't get me wrong—it performs some amazing feats along the way!

There are two types of dietary fiber: soluble fiber and insoluble fiber. Both types of fiber benefit the body in so many ways, from promoting regularity and preventing constipation to decreasing the risk for colon cancer as well as other types of cancers. In addition, fiber helps to lower cholesterol levels, reduce the risk for heart disease, and regulate blood sugar levels. As if that weren't enough, high-fiber foods and snacks can also help you to feel fuller longer after you eat, which in turn can keep you from nibbling when you shouldn't. That means fewer calories and, well, that can only mean one thing: weight loss! Fiber isn't the magic cure for weight loss, but if you replace some of those high-fat and high-sugar foods with foods that are healthy and higher in fiber, it most certainly can help.

> *FYI: A Word of Caution: It is important to increase your fiber intake gradually to avoid unpleasant side effects such as cramping, indigestion, and excess gas. Be sure to drink plenty of water and fluids daily to keep your body hydrated and to keep fiber moving through the body smoothly.*

Although fiber isn't truly considered a nutrient, it is still a very important part of a healthy and well-balanced diet, which means it is also an important part of eating for increased fertility! Fiber can be found in loads of healthy foods, including fruits, vegetables, legumes/beans, whole grains, soy foods, lentils, nuts, and seeds. How much fiber you need daily depends on your gender and your age. The recommendations by the Institute of Medicine's Food and Nutrition Board state that adult women under 50 years of age need 25 grams daily and women over 50 need 21 grams daily. And don't forget the men! Adult men under 50 years of age need 38 grams daily, and men over 50 need 30 grams daily. As long as you stick close to the recommended servings of fruits, veggies, and whole grains, and often throw in some legumes/beans, nuts and seeds, you should be able to meet your requirements.

Here are a few easy ways to increase your daily fiber:

- Start your day with a bowl of whole grain cereal, either hot or cold, and top it with sliced fresh fruit.
- Make the switch to whole wheat breads, pastas, and brown rice.
- Add barley, beans, lentils, or split peas to soups, casseroles, or stews.
- Grab a piece of fresh fruit when you get that afternoon sweet tooth.
- Don't overcook your vegetables; lightly steam them.
- Substitute part whole-wheat flour in baked goods.
- Sneak fiber into a sandwich with shredded carrots, sliced cucumbers, sliced tomato, raw spinach, and/or sprouts in between two slices of whole-wheat bread.
- Add nuts or low-fat granola to your favorite yogurt.
- Try dried fruit for something new; it is usually higher in fiber then canned or whole fruit.
- Leave the skin or peel on fruits and vegetables when possible and wash them well before eating. Most of the fiber found in fruits and vegetables is found in the skin and pulp.

FYI: *If you're checking out food labels, here is some label lingo concerning fiber:*

- *"Good Source of Fiber": 3 to less then 5 grams of fiber per serving*
- *"Contains Fiber" or "Provides Fiber": 10 to 19 percent of the daily value for fiber per serving*
- *"High Fiber," "Rich in Fiber," or "Excellent Source of Fiber": 5 grams of more of fiber (20 percent or more of the daily value for fiber) per serving*

Precious Protein

In addition to fat and carbohydrates, protein is another nutrient that adds calories to the foods we eat. And just like fat and carbs, it is essential to a well-balanced, healthy diet. Protein is found in some of the foods we eat as well as in many of our body's structures such as collagen, muscles, bones, organs, tendons, ligaments, hair, nails, teeth, and skin. Protein is used in our body to build and repair tissue, make enzymes and hormones, transport nutrients, help muscles contract, regulate body processes such as fluid balance, and the list goes on. Protein can also be used as energy if you are not getting enough in the way of carbohydrates.

Amino acids are the building blocks of protein. There are 22 amino acids; nine of them are termed *essential* because we can only get them from the foods we eat. These amino acids are strung together in different combinations and make up all of the protein our body needs to function properly. Proteins from animal sources are considered complete proteins because they contain *all* of the essential amino acids. However, if you are a vegetarian or just trying to cut back on animal proteins, take heart in knowing that eating a variety of plant foods daily will generally give you all of the amino acids your body needs to function properly.

Protein can be found in plenty of food sources, including meats, poultry, fish, nuts, seeds, peas, legumes/beans, dairy products, eggs, and soy foods. Even grains and vegetables contribute some protein to our diets. One serving of protein equals 1 ounce of meat, poultry, or fish; 1/4 cup cooked dry beans; 1 egg; 1 Tbs. of peanut butter; or 1/2 ounce of nuts. Most adults should shoot for 5 to 6 ounces of protein daily. In terms of calories, the recommendation is 10 to 35 percent of your total calories should come from protein. Keep in mind that our bodies do not store protein, so we need protein sources daily.

> *FYI: A Word of Caution regarding high-protein diets: Too much protein, especially in the form of animal protein, will most likely have negative effects on your fertility, not to mention your health and long-term weight loss efforts.*

Research has found that the foods from which we obtain the majority of our daily protein requirements may interfere with ovulation and therefore fertility. Findings indicate that getting more of your protein intake from plants (legumes/beans, nuts, seeds, peas, soy foods, peanut butter, and whole grains) and less from animal foods (lean red meat, fish, poultry, dairy products and eggs) may help to increase fertility. This doesn't mean you need to become a full-fledged vegetarian, but it might mean that throwing in a few meals a week that focus on beans, nuts, or soy and making healthier choices from your animal protein sources may provide an advantage to your fertility. Try being a little more flexible and adventurous and get your protein intake from a variety of sources. Aim for at least half of your protein servings from plant sources and the other half from healthier animal sources.

Mentioning meats, poultry, and fish

Even though a reduced intake of animal protein is often recommended, it is still a good source of protein when chosen with care. Have red meat just once or twice a week and look for words such as "loin" or "round," which will clue you in to a leaner choice. Try trimming off excess fat and leaving the skin off of poultry, and bake, broil, or grill meats, poultry, and fish to cut down on fat in cooking. Focus on keeping serving sizes under control. Keep in mind that a 3-ounce serving of meat, poultry, or fish is about the size of a deck of cards. The Dietary Guidelines for Americans recommend that all adults eat at least 8 ounces of fish weekly. Chapter 4 will discuss seafood guidelines specifically for women who are trying to become pregnant or who are already pregnant.

Doing dairy

The dairy group consists of milk, yogurt, and cheese. Fat-free and/or low-fat foods from this group are recommended. Taken together, dairy foods provide a unique package of nutrients including calcium, vitamin D, potassium, phosphorus, vitamin A, vitamin B12, riboflavin, niacin, and protein. One serving of the milk group is equal to 1 cup of milk or yogurt, 1.5 ounces natural cheese, or 2 ounces of processed cheese. The average adult should shoot for 3 cups or equivalent from this group daily.

Staying Hydrated

We have discussed most of the food groups that we need for a healthy diet and better reproductive health, but let's not forget one thing many of us tend to leave out: water! Water is essential to the body and should be your number-one beverage choice before, during, and after pregnancy. Did you know that the human body is composed of mostly water? In fact, water is present in almost every cell and every part of your body. No wonder we need it so badly! Being properly hydrated helps your body to regulate proper body temperature; transport essential nutrients and oxygen; carry waste products; cushion joints; keep skin, hair, and nails moisturized; protect body organs; assist in digestion; and prevent constipation. Not to mention the fact that being properly hydrated can help increase your energy levels and provide you with an improved sense of well-being, as well as help deliver greater endurance and stamina during physical activity.

Drinking plenty of water for good health is pretty obvious, but it can have a few fertility benefits, as well. Drinking enough water while you are trying to conceive can help increase the quality and amount of fertile cervical fluid that is essential for successful conception. It is this fluid that carries the sperm to meet the egg, so needless to say, the more you have of it the better your chances of becoming pregnant. Not only is water important to conception but it is also a necessity during pregnancy. Because most of us don't know we are pregnant right away, drinking lots of water during the TTC phase is a good idea. Plus, by getting into the good habit of drinking plenty of water for TTC and pregnancy, you have an added bonus of adopting a good healthy habit for life.

For most adults, the goal should be anywhere between 8 to 12 cups per day, depending on your size, the environment, and your activity level. If you haven't been much of a water drinker up to this point, you may notice some extra trips to the bathroom at first; as your body becomes accustomed to the additional fluid intake, that will decrease somewhat. If your main excuse for not drinking water is not liking the taste, not that there is much flavor, try adding the juice from a fresh lemon or lime.

Already feeling thirsty? Then you are already on your way to dehydration. Our bodies do not store water, so you need to continually replace it. Keep a water bottle with you so you can drink from it often throughout the day. What better way to quench your thirst than a beverage that contains *zero* calories and does more then its share for our health?

Nutrition Rules to Live By

To sum it up a bit, here are some important fertility-friendly nutrition rules to live by:

- Consume a good balance of fats, carbs, and protein each day and shoot for the recommended goals for each.

- Choose healthier fats. Out with the saturated and trans fats, and in with the monounsaturated, polyunsaturated, and omega-3 fats.

- Choose more complex carbohydrates and whole grains and limit refined grains and sugary foods.

- Eat plenty of fruits and vegetables with an array of varieties and colors.

- Add more plant proteins to your diet and be sure that the animal proteins you choose are leaner versions.

- Drink plenty of water throughout the day.

- Make changes to your diet slowly and keep in mind that you don't have to be perfect all the time. Eating healthily most of the time will help get you the results you are looking for.

Chapter 4

Everything You Always Wanted to Ask a Dietitian About Trying to Conceive

? Do I need to avoid fish when I am trying to conceive?

If you are a woman who might become pregnant, is already pregnant, or is nursing, there are a few rules to follow when it comes to eating fish. If you have young children at home, listen up, because they are a part of this group, as well. If you are trying to conceive or are in any of the groups mentioned previously, you don't need to steer completely clear of fish and shellfish, but there are safety guidelines that you should follow. Fish and shellfish should be part of a healthy diet and contain high quality protein, loads of essential nutrients such as B vitamins and those very beneficial omega-3 fats (specifically DHA and EPA) that we discussed in Chapter 3. Fish and shellfish are low in saturated fats and cholesterol. Fatty fish, and that is "good" fat, are good sources of vitamin A and vitamin D as well as other essential nutrients that are vital for a developing baby and a healthy pregnancy.

The problem is that even though fish and shellfish are full of healthy stuff, certain species contain traces of mercury, some more then others. For most people this doesn't pose a health problem, but for a few select groups of people, such as the ones mentioned previously, it can. Our body easily absorbs the mercury found in fish and shellfish and can store it for months. During pregnancy, the mercury you consume can also cross the placenta to the fetus. Being exposed to higher levels of mercury may harm the fetus, specifically, the developing nervous system and brain (which will affect things like memory, attention, language, motor skills, and possibly vision).

Experts still have not completely agreed on how much mercury is actually harmful, but it is a good idea for the more vulnerable groups of people to avoid fish that is high in mercury and limit, though by no means eliminate, other fish and shellfish in the diet. Fish and shellfish provide far too many essential nutrients to give them up totally, and most experts agree that the benefits of eating fish probably outweigh the risks. Nonetheless, the FDA and EPA have developed specific guidelines for pregnant women, women of childbearing age, nursing moms, and young children.

By following these safety guidelines, people at risk can still enjoy adding fish and shellfish to their diet while reducing harmful exposure to too much mercury.

- Avoid eating shark, swordfish, king mackerel, and tilefish altogether: all of these species contain high levels of mercury.

- Eat up to 12 ounces (about two average meals) per week of a variety of fish and shellfish that contain lower mercury content. The five most commonly eaten fish that are low in mercury are shrimp, canned light tuna, salmon, pollock, and catfish, though you don't need to stick to just these varieties. Albacore (white) tuna contains more mercury than canned light tuna. Do not eat more then 6 ounces of albacore tuna per week as part of your 12 ounces of fish or shellfish per week.

- If you love to fish, check with your local advisories about the safety of the fish you catch in local lakes, rivers, and coastal areas. If you cannot find any information on the fish you catch, make it a rule of thumb to eat no more then 6 ounces of the fish you catch from local waters and not consume any other fish or shellfish that week.

- These same recommendations should be used when feeding fish to young children, but serve smaller portions.

- For more information visit: *www.epa.gov/ost/fish*.

So why is it that women of childbearing age need to be concerned about the mercury content in fish and shellfish? Firstly, you don't always realize you are pregnant right away and it can take weeks to be aware of that. Secondly, if you eat a lot of fish that is high in mercury, it will accumulate in your bloodstream through time. Mercury is removed from the body naturally, but it can take a lot of time, even up to a year, before levels drop significantly. So once you become pregnant, even if you stop eating fish high in mercury, there may be enough accumulated in your bloodstream to cause concern.

The bottom line is that the recommendation of most experts, including the American Heart Association, to reap the benefits of omega-3 fatty acids is to eat two servings of fish per week. At 3 to 4 ounces per serving that is well below the FDA and EPA's safe limit of 12 ounces per week. Eating a variety of fish and following these recommendations and precautions will ensure that you can still be able to enjoy fish, feel safe, and enjoy all of its healthy benefits.

⟨?⟩ How can I get omega-3 fat without eating fish?

If you are not a fish eater but want those healthy omega-3 fats in your diet, there are other ways to get it. Omega-3 fatty acids can also be found in a variety of plant foods such as dark green leafy vegetables, walnuts, soybeans, ground flaxseeds, pumpkin seeds, and numerous nut oils in the form of ALA (alpha linolenic acid). The body is able to covert ALA into EPA and DHA. The process isn't 100-percent efficient and only a small amount of ALA is actually converted to EPA and DHA, so you need to eat quite a bit of these foods to produce enough EPA and DHA to provide all of the health benefits.

Although most experts recommend increasing your consumption of omega-3 fats through whole foods that naturally provide the fat, you can now find foods fortified with omega-3 fats as well as fish oil supplements that supply this healthy fat. Fortified foods don't contain omega-3 naturally; instead, the fat is added and they are fortified with it. These foods include certains kinds of milk, eggs, yogurt, peanut butter, bread, margarine, and pasta. These fortified foods usually contain very little of this healthy fat, so you would need to eat a lot of them to get close to what is recommended. Additional omega-3 fatty acids found in these foods aren't harmful but you shouldn't completely substitute these "functional foods" for ones that naturally contain omega-3 fats. If you are not sure how much omega-3 fat or which type (ALA, EPA, or DHA) is in there, be sure to check the label.

As far as fish oil supplements go, they are not always the magic pills that some believe; in fact, some experts will tell you that supplements may not be the best idea. They argue that it might be more than just the omega-3 fatty acids found in fish that contribute to its overall health benefits, and that wouldn't be found in fish oil supplements alone. Still others believe that fish oil supplements can be quite beneficial, especially for those people who do not eat fish. If you are taking a supplement you need to read labels closely. Most of the fish oil supplements on the market do provide EPA and DHA and are virtually free of mercury, although contaminants such as mercury and PCBs can accumulate in fish oil just as they do in fish, so look for supplements made from purified fish oil to be on the safe side. Use only reputable brands that are pharmaceutical grade, which means it has met freshness and purity standards and often contain a higher potency of EPA and DHA in a single capsule. If you decide that fish oil supplements are the way to go, be warned that taking too much, particularly more than what is recommended, can increase your risk of bleeding and bruising, which isn't likely to happen from foods.

FYI: It is highly recommended that you consult with your healthcare provider before taking a fish oil supplement or any supplement, especially if you have a medical condition, are taking prescription medications, have any food allergies, are pregnant or trying to become pregnant. Always let your doctor know if you are taking fish oil supplements because they inhibit blood clotting and may cause other issues for some people.

The amount of fish oil listed on the label of a fish oil supplement can sometimes be misleading. Just because a supplement lists 1 gram or 1,000 mg of fish oil doesn't mean it is all coming from omega-3 fats. The amount of EPA and DHA is the most important component because this is the true indicator of the amount of healthy omega-3 fats in the supplement. For example, if the label states that the 1,000 mg fish oil supplement contains 250 mg of EPA and 250 mg of DHA, it has a total of 500 mg of omega-3 fats, not 1,000 mg. So instead of looking for total fish oil content in the capsule, look for the amount of EPA and DHA per serving.

The bottom line is that omega-3 fats have health and possibly fertility benefits, but as with the other healthy fats, rather than being an addition to your diet, they should replace the unhealthy fats. If fish is not your favorite food, try to get what you need with a combination of ALA foods, fortified foods, and supplements.

? Do I have to give up my coffee?

- You can take a deep breath and relax. You don't need to give up all of your coffee and other favorite caffeine-containing foods and beverages. But—and there is always a "but"—you should keep them in check and consume them in moderate amounts if you are trying to conceive.

- Caffeine, an ingredient found in coffee, tea, soft drinks, energy drinks, chocolate drinks and even some foods such as chocolate, acts as a stimulant as well as a diuretic. Stimulants rev up your central nervous system, increasing your heart rate, keeping you awake, and making you jittery. Diuretics stimulate urination and can affect the fluid levels in your body by reducing them at a time when you need to be properly hydrated. Some studies have found that high levels of caffeine intake can quite possibly have a negative impact on fertility. For women who are pregnant studies have shown that caffeine in amounts more than 200 milligrams (mg) per day (about 12 ounces of brewed coffee or 2 small cups) may cause miscarriages and possibly slow the growth of a developing fetus. Not to mention that too much caffeine can reduce the absorption of calcium and iron in the body, two essential nutrients during pregnancy. Therefore it only makes sense that if you are actively trying to conceive, err on the side of caution and make every effort to stay under the 200 mg limit.

- If you are only a light coffee drinker and don't drink much in the way of tea or soft drinks, you may already be at a safe limit. If you are a big caffeine drinker, from coffee or any other caffeine-containing food or beverage, you should probably trim back a bit. Wean yourself slowly and don't go cold turkey so that you can avoid withdrawal symptoms such as headaches, irritability, trouble concentrating, and fatigue. For example, start by switching to half decaf and half caffeinated coffee. Begin slowly cutting back on the number of cups of coffee or caffeine-containing beverages you drink. Keep in mind how much caffeine is in coffee, as stated previously, and that caffeinated soft drinks contain around 35 to 45 mg per can; tea, about 40 to 60 mg per cup; and energy drinks, a whopping 80 mg per can. There are even some over-the-counter medications such as allergy drugs or migraine medicines that can also contain caffeine.

Can't seem to give up that afternoon cup of coffee or soft drink? Substitute it with a cold glass of water and you can kill two birds with one stone! If doing without makes you feel tired in the afternoon, take a walk around the office or eat a healthy snack for a healthier pick-me-up instead! Once you have become accustomed to life with only moderate caffeine you will never know the difference.

? *Is it okay to drink diet soft drinks?*

That daily habit of drinking diet soft drinks is really just a habit full of empty calories—well, not even calories, just empty. They offer absolutely no nutritional benefits and can fill you up, keeping you from drinking or consuming healthier foods that *do* offer nutritional benefits. Diet soft drinks may have less caffeine than a cup of coffee, but they also contain artificial sweeteners such as aspartame, acesulfame-K, and saccharin in place of sugar. Although the jury still seems to be out on this one, at this point the general consensus is that aspartame (also known as Nutrasweet) and acesulfame-K are safe to consume in moderation while trying to conceive and during pregnancy. However, many experts have found that saccharin can cross the placenta during pregnancy, so it is usually the one sweetener doctors will warn patients about consuming during pregnancy. The bottom line is that if you must drink diet soft drinks or use artificial sweeteners in other beverages, do so in moderation. But consider kicking the habit now and switching to a beverage that is full of nutrition and which will benefit conception as well as a healthy pregnancy and baby.

If you are confused as to what to use to sweeten your coffee or tea, real sugar in small amounts is always an option. It won't leave you wondering about possible side effects now or down the road. If you are concerned about the safety of artificial sweeteners you are currently using, speak with your healthcare provider.

Don't mistakenly think that a switch from diet soft drinks to regular will do you any good! Regular soft drinks are just as full of empty calories. On average, a 12-ounce soft drink can deliver 150 to 200 empty calories and a whopping nine to 11 teaspoons of pure sugar. That amount of sugar will cause spikes in both blood sugar and insulin and, in the long term, cause weight gain, both of which can make becoming pregnant difficult. Substitute healthy beverages such as water, milk, and/or 100-percent juice for your diet or regular soft drinks.

? *Can I drink alcohol?*

There is no doubt that heavy drinking and/or alcohol abuse can be harmful to many aspects of life, including fertility. Moderate alcohol intake, on the other hand, comes with a bit of controversy. By moderate drinking we are talking about one drink a day for women and two per day for men. A drink is a 12-ounce beer, 5-ounce glass of wine, or a 1.5 ounce shot of liquor. Some experts will warn you that any alcohol intake while trying to conceive or during pregnancy can cause harm, whereas others will say that an occasional drink is fine. The truth is that experts have not yet concluded what a safe level of alcohol intake for women who are pregnant or trying to conceive is. Either way, if you are trying to conceive, it is probably a good idea to begin cutting way back and to eventually quit. If you are actively timing things out and you know you are in the 2-week wait period from ovulation to your menstrual cycle, you will most definitely want to do more then cut back. If you are not timing things out and usually are not sure where you are in your cycle, you may want to seriously consider staying away from alcohol. Birth defects that are associated with prenatal alcohol exposure can occur in the first 8 weeks of pregnancy; many women don't even know they are pregnant at that point. In addition, some research has shown that even a moderate amount of alcohol may possibly increase your chances of miscarriage in those early weeks when you don't even know you are expecting.

Women shouldn't be drinking their mocktails (non-alcoholic cocktails) alone! If you are actively trying to conceive, your partner should also refrain or at least cut back on the alcohol, as too much alcohol for men can damage sperm as well as reduce the quantity sperm.

? Are there any specific foods that will help me get pregnant?

That would most definitely be a good thing if we could eat certain foods that would help us get pregnant. Unfortunately there are no individual foods that have been scientifically proven to increase your chances of conception. It is best to stick with what *is* known, and that is an overall healthier and well-balanced diet and lifestyle. This we know can help increase your chances of conceiving. It will do a lot more for you in general than just trying to eat specific foods.

A registered dietitian can help you review your current dietary intake to pinpoint what might be lacking and to help you fill those voids by eating a healthier diet in general. Chapter 7 will touch on some of the popular unproven diet and/or food remedies for fertility.

? Will eating organic foods help?

Currently there is no scientific evidence that consuming organic foods will definitely help you get pregnant more quickly or increase your fertility, but there is quite a bit of speculation swirling around this topic. More seems to be known about these foods being a healthier option during pregnancy therefore it isn't a bad idea to begin thinking of ways to go organic while trying to conceive. Organic produce isn't necessarily more nutritious than conventional produce. However, organically grown fruit and vegetables will likely be fairly close to pesticide free as possible, and for animal foods such as meats and dairy products, the animals are not treated with antibiotics or growth hormones or given feed made from animal byproducts. The main idea is that there is no downside to going organic but at this point the jury is still out on it being the magic bullet on the road to successful conception. In fact, potentially there can be a benefit to introducing organic foods into your daily diet.

Most large chain grocery stores are stocked with organic meats, dairy foods, produce, and even packaged foods. The problem for most people is that organic foods can be somewhat more expensive than non-organic foods, and that may make it difficult for you to add these foods to your weekly grocery list. The solution is to focus just on the foods that carry the heaviest amounts of pesticides, additives, and hormones. According to the Environmental Working Group, you can reduce your intake of these things quite a bit by eating organic when it comes to the most contaminated foods. They have developed a list of the worst produce offenders, which they call the "Dirty Dozen" even though they have added a few since the title was given. If you can't go all organic, at least consider going organic with the produce foods on this list, which can help you to lower your intake of potentially dangerous chemical additives. Besides produce, keep in mind that milk, meat, and even coffee can be high on the contaminated foods list.

The "Dirty Dozen":

- Apples
- Blueberries
- Cherries
- Grapes (imported)
- Nectarines
- Peaches
- Strawberries
- Bell peppers
- Potatoes
- Kale
- Spinach
- Celery

No need to buy organic with these foods:

- Bananas
- Kiwis
- Mangos
- Papayas
- Pineapples
- Watermelon
- Cantaloupe (domestic)
- Asparagus
- Avocado
- Broccoli
- Sweet corn
- Onions
- Sweet peas
- Cabbage
- Eggplant
- Tomatos
- Sweet potato

For a full list of best to worst produce, go to: *www.foodnews. org/fulllist.php.*

> *FYI: If you are looking for a food that is 100-percent organic, you need to look for the words "100% Organic" on the label. If the food bears a USDA Organic label, it is produced and processed according to USDA standards and contains at least 95 percent of ingredients that are organically produced. The phrase "Made with organic ingredients" means the product contains at least 70 percent organic ingredients. Don't fall for the labels "Natural," "All Natural," "Free-Range," or "Hormone-free," as none of these mean organic.*

Another option for lowering your intake of pesticides and additives is to visit the local farmer markets in your area. Small local farms tend to be less aggressive than large farms when it comes to spraying their produce with chemicals. Not only will you be buying fresher and healthier fruits and vegetables, but you will be supporting your local economy and helping out the environment.

Always wash all fresh fruits and vegetables. If they are not organic, be sure to wash them very thoroughly to reduce the amount of dirt and bacteria. For produce that has skin that you will eat, such as apples, potatoes, or cucumbers, use a small scrub brush to clean them well. If you are still concerned about pesticides, peel your fruits and vegetables and trim outer leaves of green leafy vegetables in addition to washing them. Keep in mind that by peeling some fruits and vegetables, you may be reducing the amount of nutrients and fiber.

The Environmental Working Group revises their lists yearly, so check back often: *www.foodnews.org.*

? Will a vegetarian diet hurt my chances of becoming pregnant?

Absolutely not! Vegetarians, including vegans who eat absolutely *no* animal products at all, get pregnant all the time and have healthy pregnancies and babies. However, just as you would with a regular diet, you need to be more conscious of what you are eating when you are trying to conceive. You need to look at your current vegetarian diet and ensure it is well-balanced, and that means plenty of protein, complex carbohydrates, and healthy fats as well as other essential nutrients. If you include dairy foods, eggs, and fish, you probably will be fine as long as you balance those foods with plenty of fruits, vegetables, nuts/seeds, legumes, and whole grains. If you are a vegan, it can become a bit more challenging. You will need to ensure you are getting nutrients important to good reproductive health, such as zinc and vitamin B12, which are usually found in animal foods. You may need to include foods such as potatoes with the skin on (scrubbed well, of course), wheat germ, black-eyed peas, oatmeal, and fortified foods such as some cereals. Iron can be another dicey nutrient that vegans may fall short on. Look to plant foods such as spinach, legumes, lentils, and oats to fill your quota. On the plus side, vegetarians usually get their allowance of the all-important vitamin, folate, and then some, even more than meat eaters do, as folate is found in many plant foods.

Taking a prenatal vitamin, which you should be doing anyway, will help to fill in the gaps where you're falling short. However, don't use your prenatal supplement to take the place of foods or food groups. Try to get in as many nutrients as possible through food sources and use the supplement to do just that—supplement your diet! Because being a vegetarian, especially a vegan, can make consuming a fertility-friendly diet a bit more challenging, it is a good idea to sit down with a registered dietitian who can analyze your current dietary intake and pinpoint the areas where you may be lacking. A dietitian can help you plan a diet that is right for you and perfect for trying to conceive!

? Should I avoid soy and soy foods?

Soy is another controversial subject when it comes to a fertility-friendly diet. Soy products are everywhere these days in the form of soymilk, soy yogurt, soy cheese, soybeans, tofu, tempeh, soy hot dogs, tofu turkey, and the list goes on. For vegetarians, especially, it can be a popular food choice because it is a high-quality protein source. Even for those who are not vegetarians, soy has been touted as a miracle food full of protein, calcium, and other healthy nutrients. Some headlines read that soy products can help lower cholesterol, decrease hot flashes in menopausal women, and prevent breast and prostate cancer. Others read that soy products could increase your risk for breast and prostate cancers. Very confusing! The culprit in all the confusion seems to be the phytoestrogens found in soy foods. These phytoestrogens appear to mimic the estrogen in the body, and whether that suppresses or promotes problems such as cancer and infertility is uncertain. This uncertainty is the best reason to go easy on the soy, and that goes for men as well as women. This is not to say that you should completely eliminate these foods from your diet, but you shouldn't overdo it, either. In fact, occasionally swapping an animal protein source such as meat for a plant-based protein source such as soy can work in your favor. Soy foods in a varied diet can offer healthy alternative proteins that are low in saturated fat and cholesterol-free. Focus on eating whole soy foods. Research has shown that whole soy foods generally do not contribute to the recurrence of breast and prostate cancer. Whole soy foods include foods such as miso, tempeh, tofu, soybeans, soy nuts, soymilk, and soy yogurt. Avoid heavily processed soy foods such as soy protein isolate, soy protein concentrate, hydrolyzed soy protein, and texturized soy protein (TSP), and soy supplements. Read the labels of the soy foods you choose so that you can be sure you know what you are eating. Want to take it a step further? Opt for organic whole soy products, which are available at most of the larger chain grocery stores. Keep in mind that soy is a common source of food sensitivity for both children and adults.

The bottom line is that if you are a big soy eater and you are trying to conceive, female or male, you should not only consider cutting back but also double checking the soy foods you do eat to ensure they don't include large amounts of processed soy. If you are concerned about the amount of soy you currently consume or you are not sure what is a safe level for you, speak with your healthcare provider and/or a registered dietitian. If you are a vegetarian and are unsure how to include more protein while cutting back on soy, speak to a dietitian for individual diet recommendations.

? Is it okay to diet if I'm trying to conceive?

We already know that being overweight can hurt your chances of becoming pregnant. And we know that a modest weight loss toward your healthy weight can help to improve those chances. If possible, your best bet is to lose some of your excess weight before you begin your journey of trying to conceive by eating more healthily and exercising. You most definitely do not want to diet in an extreme way at any time, but especially when you are trying to conceive. Slow and steady weight loss is what you are after. Changing lifestyle habits for good is the key to a weight loss you can maintain for life. Check back to Chapter 2 for more information on the best way to lose weight and maintain a healthy weight for increased fertility.

? Should I take mega doses of vitamins?

No, you definitely do not want to go supplement crazy when you are trying to conceive, and you don't want to put your baby at risk if you become pregnant. Certain vitamins such as A, D, E and K are fat-soluble vitamins that can be stored in the body and build up to toxic levels. For example, too much vitamin A (as preformed vitamin A and not as beta-carotene) can actually cause birth defects. The Institute of Medicine considers 3,000 mcg (10,000 IU) to be the maximum upper level of preformed vitamin A that you should get from a combination of supplements, foods, and fortified foods each day. Women under 19 years of age should get no more then 2,800 mcg (9,240 IU).

Water-soluble vitamins, on the other hand, such as the B vitamins and vitamin C, are not stored in the body, but mega doses can still cause problems. Stick with supplements that stay within 100 percent of the recommended daily allowances and couple that with a healthy well-balanced diet to get what you need. If you are trying to conceive, either take a prenatal vitamin/mineral supplement that will supply all you need or take a multivitamin with at least 400 mcg of folic acid. Speak with your healthcare provider about which supplement will meet your individual needs.

? Does my male partner need to watch his nutritional intake?

It takes two to tango when you are trying to become pregnant, and that means that both of you need to watch your nutritional intake and choose a healthier lifestyle. Men need to ensure they are getting all of the essential vitamins and minerals they need to be in top form for the job. The lifestyle choices that your partner makes can, without a doubt, affect your chances for conception. The sooner your man begins a healthier lifestyle, the better, so just as *you* are following the advice in this book toward a healthier diet and overall healthier lifestyle, make sure you take your partner along for the ride!

A few tips for men:

- Eat plenty of fruits and vegetables. Studies have shown that men who consume at least five or more servings per day of a variety of brightly colored produce are more fertile then men who don't.

- Just as recommended for women follow the Dietary Guidelines for Americans and MyPlate to help you consume a healthy, well-balanced diet daily.

- Include plenty of omega-3 fats, as discussed previously, in your daily diet.

- Even though you may be eating right, it is good idea to take a daily multivitamin that supplies around 100 percent of essential vitamins and minerals and contains zinc and selenium. Although many nutrients are essential for good fertility health, zinc and selenium specifically help aid in the development of healthy sperm.

- Moderate your caffeine intake.

- Cut back on alcohol if you drink. An occasional drink is generally considered safe, but too much can lower sperm counts and raise the number of abnormal sperm.

- Live an active lifestyle and drink plenty of water.

Chapter 5

Conception-Welcoming Nutrients for Her and Him

Now that the macronutrients in your diet (protein, carbohydrates, and fats) are in better balance, it is time to take a closer look at the micronutrients (vitamins and minerals). Don't let the "micro" part fool you! They are just as important and mighty as macronutrients. All vitamins and minerals are essential to good health, but it is how they synergistically work together that creates their powerful punch in the conception arena! Don't wait until you are pregnant to start including these valuable nutrients in your daily diet. That may just be too late!

Take into account that following a healthy and well-balanced diet along with taking a daily multivitamin or prenatal vitamin/ mineral supplement can help ensure you are getting all you need. There is no need to start taking supplements for individual vitamins and/or minerals unless prescribed by your healthcare provider. In fact, doing so can upset the balance and do more harm than good. Each micronutrient contributes a little something, but a few stand out as contributing a little something extra to the whole baby-making process and pregnancy.

Featuring Folic Acid

Folic acid is a B vitamin but it is no ordinary B vitamin. It is one that takes center stage while you are trying to conceive and once you become pregnant. And there is good reason for that. Getting the recommended daily amount of folic acid can help reduce the risk of birth defects of the brain and spine (called *neural tube defects*) such as spina bifida, as well as other types of birth defects. You must have plenty of folic acid stores available before you become pregnant to prevent these types of birth defects because many of them develop during the first month of pregnancy. In addition to helping to prevent birth defects, folic acid may also help lower your risk of experiencing a premature delivery once you become pregnant.

Folic acid is essential for cell division, red blood cell production, and production of our DNA (our genetic make-up). During pregnancy the reproduction of DNA is fast and furious, so it is no wonder that folic acid appears to deal firsthand with the start of a pregnancy and the prevention of birth defects. Folic acid is vital not only in the months preceding conception and the first month of pregnancy but also throughout your entire pregnancy.

? How much is needed?

Terminology can get confusing when it comes to this B vitamin. It can be called folic acid or folate. To put it simply, folate is the form that is naturally found in some foods. Folic acid, on the other hand, is the man-made or synthetic form of folate. It is folic acid that is found in supplements such as prenatals and in fortified foods. Surprisingly, folic acid is more readily absorbed and more easily used by the body then folate, the natural form. In addition, cooking and storage of foods can many times destroy some of the folate that a food contains.

The Dietary Reference Intake (DRI), the recommendations set by the government, for folate is 400 micrograms (mcg) daily for women of childbearing age. Once a woman becomes pregnant, that recommendation jumps to 600 mcg daily.

FYI: The DRI is expressed as not folate or folic acid but as Dietary Folate Equivalents (DFE's). This was developed to account for the differences in absorption of folate and folic acid.

1 DFE = 1 mcg food folate = 0.6 mcg folic acid from supplements and fortified foods

---

Even with the difference in absorption, most experts recommend that women of childbearing age get 400 to 800 mcg of folic acid daily. A general multivitamin/mineral supplement will usually provide 400 mcg of folic acid, whereas prenatal supplements generally provide more. More is sometimes better *but* only for specific groups of women. Women who have had a baby with a birth defect of the brain or spine and want to conceive again may need much more than the recommended dose to help lower their risk of having another baby with these birth defects. Women who have a family member with spina bifida or have it themselves will need a higher level of folic acid then what is generally recommended if they are trying to conceive and/or are of childbearing age. Some prescription medications and/or health conditions may increase your need for folic acid, as well. These higher levels of folic acid need to be prescribed by your healthcare provider. Do not try to increase your folic acid by taking more of your prenatal or multivitamin supplement then what is recommended. This can cause you to get too much of other vitamins and minerals that are included in your supplement. You can't get too much folate from foods that naturally contain it, but you can get too much folic acid from supplements so be aware of how much you are taking. Too much folic acid can mask a vitamin B12 deficiency, and that can lead to health problems such as nerve damage. Unless your healthcare provider instructs you otherwise, do not consume more then 1,000 mcg of folic acid daily.

Men need folic acid, too. Not getting enough can lead to low sperm quality and possible birth defects. Taking a daily multivitamin/mineral supplement and eating fortified foods such as breakfast cereals as well as foods naturally containing folate such as leafy greens, legumes, and orange juice will help supplement any extra you might need. Men actually need the same amount as women, 400 mcg daily.

> FYI: Take your multivitamin/mineral or prenatal supplement with food to increase the absorption of vitamins such as folic acid.

Food sources

Because a little extra folic acid might just aid in conception, don't rely on supplementation alone but also look to the foods you eat, including both fortified foods and foods that naturally contain folate. If you play your cards right you can technically get all the folate you need from food alone, though a supplement will ensure that. Folic acid can be found in and is actually required by the FDA to be in fortified grain foods such as cereals, breads, rice, and pastas. The term "fortified" means that folic acid is added to foods that do not already contain folate. In addition to fortified foods, there are plenty of foods that naturally contain folate. The following make for some good choices when adding folic acid and folate to your diet:

- Leafy green vegetables
- Whole-wheat bread
- Whole-grain fortified cereals
- Brown rice
- Whole-wheat pasta
- Citrus fruit and juices
- Broccoli
- Asparagus
- Legumes/dried beans/peas
- Lentils

Caring About Calcium

Calcium is an important mineral that you should care about throughout your life. Getting enough calcium, especially in your younger years is vital to good bone health. And it is just as important to stock up on calcium while you are trying to conceive and before you become pregnant. Calcium is essential for strong, healthy bones and teeth and facilitates muscle contractions, your heartbeat, normal nerve function, and blood clotting. Calcium is believed to help reduce the risk of high blood pressure, and for women who suffer with premenstrual syndrome, or PMS, consuming enough calcium can help to alleviate some of those troublesome symptoms.

Because a baby's teeth form so early during pregnancy, it is a smart idea to ensure you are getting plenty of calcium while you are trying to conceive. The baby will take what he/she needs from your own calcium stores, so if you don't have enough stored up, that can leave you short and with problems down the road, such as osteoporosis. If you tend to skimp on the dairy foods, keep in mind that not only does plenty of calcium help strengthen your baby-to-be's developing teeth and bones, but it also plays a role in the development of his or her heart, muscles, and nerves.

⍰ *How much is needed?*

The DRI for most women of childbearing age, 19 to 50 years of age, is 1,000 mg of calcium daily. That same amount goes for women of the same age who might be pregnant or who are breastfeeding as well as for men. Consuming plenty of calcium-rich foods daily can ensure you are getting what you need. But if you are not sure you are getting enough calcium in your daily diet, you may want to consider a calcium supplement to be sure you are hitting your goal. Most prenatal and multivitamin/mineral supplements don't contain a whole lot of calcium, so it is best not to rely on them for additional calcium. There is aactually a reason for this: Most prenatals are higher in iron and unfortunately iron and calcium don't do well together. Calcium can bind to iron and interfere with the absorption of both. If you do take a calcium supplement, it is best to take it at a different time of day then your prenatal supplement.

One of the key factors when trying to decide which calcium supplement to buy is the amount of *elemental calcium* it contains. This term refers to the calcium in the supplement that is available for your body to absorb and use. Check the label of the supplement to find out how much elemental calcium the product actually contains. The elemental calcium should be listed in milligrams according to serving size, which is usually one or two tablets. If the supplement label states it contains 500 mg of calcium carbonate, it may only provide 200 mg of elemental calcium, so your supplement is only providing 200 mg of calcium and not 500 mg. As with all supplements, more is not always better. Do not consume more then 2,500 mg of elemental calcium daily, which is the Upper Tolerable Limit set by the government for adults 19 to 50 years of age.

Calcium in supplements usually comes bound to another element; citrate or carbonate are two of the most absorbable forms. Carbonate supplements are the most popular on the market but need to be taken with food for maximum absorption. Citrate can be taken with or without food, but these supplements tend to contain less elemental calcium then carbonate supplements.

Also important in achieving maximum benefit from a calcium supplement is the addition of magnesium and/or vitamin D, which are both essential in assisting with the absorption of calcium in the body. Look for one or both of these added nutrients. Natural sources of calcium, such as milk, are fortified with vitamin D for just that reason. Calcium supplements are absorbed most efficiently when taken in amounts of somewhere between 500 and 600 mg at one time. If you take 1,000 mg daily, split it into at least two doses over the course of the day. Keep in mind that some health conditions and/or prescription medications can affect the use of calcium supplements. Speak with your healthcare provider concerning the daily amount of calcium that you should be taking. Don't rely completely on calcium supplements to provide all the calcium your body needs. They should only be used to supplement a diet full of calcium-rich foods.

Food sources

Dairy foods are what usually come to mind when it comes to getting your fill of calcium. The Dietary Guidelines for Americans urge adults to consume at least 3 cups daily of milk and milk products or other dairy-rich foods, with one serving equaling 1 cup of milk, 1 cup of yogurt, or 1.5 ounces of cheese. But keep in mind there are other foods that can help to fulfill your daily needs. For those people who are lactose intolerant and cannot handle most dairy foods, this is an important bit of information. The following is a list of foods you can use to fill up on calcium:

- Milk
- Cheese
- Yogurt
- Calcium-fortified orange juice
- Calcium-fortified soy milk
- Calcium-fortified, lactose-free milk (for those who are lactose intolerant)
- Fortified cereals and oatmeal
- Sardines
- Salmon, canned, with bones
- Dark green leafy vegetables
- Tofu
- Soybeans
- Sesame seeds
- Almonds

Adding Iron

There is a good reason we need iron in our diets. When you get that friendly visit every month, a good majority of your iron stores are depleted by the blood you lose. If your menstrual flow is heavy, you will lose even more iron. Ensuring you have adequate iron stores before conceiving will give your body a chance to replenish those stores before they are needed during pregnancy. During pregnancy, your need for iron goes even higher to match your increase in blood volume. Making sure you are getting plenty of iron now will also lower your risk for iron-deficiency anemia during pregnancy. Your body will take care of the baby's iron needs first, which can leave you short if you are not getting enough, which in turn can lead to anemia, or low iron levels. Why do we need iron? Iron helps carry oxygen in your blood from your lungs to every cell in your body, it helps in brain development, and helps to support a healthy immune system. For women who are trying to conceive, there are even more reasons to pump up the iron levels. Researchers have found that women who have adequate iron stores seem to have a higher fertility rate then those who are iron deficient. Even a mild iron deficiency, which probably wouldn't be diagnosed as actual anemia, can still affect ovulation, making it more difficult to become pregnant. Women who have iron-deficiency anemia tend to have disruptions to their menstrual cycle, which, as we all know, doesn't do much for successful conception.

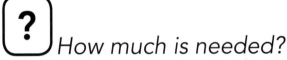

How much is needed?

Women need about 18 mg of iron daily. Once you are pregnant your need for iron shoots up to 27 mg to support the pregnancy and baby. If you are eating a healthy, well-balanced diet and taking a prenatal supplement, you shouldn't have an issue with your iron intake. However, if a blood test reveals that you are lacking iron, stemming from diet or health reasons, and you need more than your diet can provide, your healthcare provider may prescribe a supplement. Because most women do not need additional iron, do not go ahead with supplementation without speaking to your healthcare provider first. Because men do not go through a monthly menstrual cycle, their iron needs are much lower than they are for women. Men older then 19 years of age need 8 mg daily.

Food Sources

Most of us get plenty of iron in our diet. However, it is the food source the iron comes from that dictates how easily it will be absorbed into and used by the body. There are two forms of iron. *Heme iron* is the form of iron found in animal foods and is much more absorbable then the iron found in plant foods, known as *non-heme iron*. That doesn't mean that you should only get iron from animal foods. But you should try to get plenty of iron from a variety of foods. In fact, the absorption of non-heme iron can be improved when you consume it with a heme source of iron in the same meal. Coupling your iron-rich plant foods with a vitamin C source can pump up its absorption, as well. So try a glass of OJ with your morning oatmeal, dice up tomatoes to add to your beans, and add sliced strawberries to your spinach salad.

Here is a list of some iron-rich foods, including heme and non-heme sources:

- Lean red meat, poultry, and pork
- Seafood (clams, oysters, mussels, shrimp, sardines)
- Fortified breakfast cereals
- Spinach and other dark green leafy vegetables
- Beans (red kidney beans, lima beans)
- Soybean nuts
- Pumpkin seeds
- Egg yolk
- Dried fruits (raisins, prunes, apricots)
- Wheat bran

Discovering Choline

Choline may be one of those vitamins you rarely hear about but it can be very important, especially during pregnancy. Choline is a water-soluble vitamin that is included in the B-complex group and is essential for good health and disease prevention. Choline, like folate, is essential for the normal functioning of all of the body's cells, including brain and nerve function, liver metabolism, and the tranport of nutrients inside the body. Choline becomes even more important during pregnancy and breastfeeding, as it is essential for brain and memory development in the fetus and newborn and can quite possibly reduce the risk of certain neural tube birth defects. In addition, preliminary evidence appears promising that choline may help reduce the risk of heart disease, breast cancer, dementia, and Alzheimer's disease, and may even possess anti-inflammatory properties.

? How much is needed?

Because many women don't know they are pregnant until after the fact, it is important to get enough choline daily while you are trying to conceive. Once you become pregnant and/or are breastfeeding, your body's need for choline rises even higher because there is a high rate of transfer of choline from the mother to the fetus and from the mother to the baby during breastfeeding. The Adequate Intake (AI) levels for choline are 425 mg daily for women 19 years and older, and 550 mg for men 19 years and older. AI for pregnant women is slightly higher at 450 mg daily, and breastfeeding women should get 550 mg daily.

Food sources

Even though our body does take care of producing some choline, it unfortunately isn't enough to meet our daily needs. Regularly eating foods that are naturally rich in choline is your best way to make sure you are getting what your body requires. Foods rich in choline include beef and chicken liver, egg yolk, soybeans, beef, milk, wheat germ, cauliflower, bananas, oranges, lentils, oats, flaxseeds, whole-wheat bread, peanut butter, and peanuts.

Other Essential Nutrients

We have discussed some very important nutrients to consider when you are trying to conceive. But that isn't the last of them! There are plenty more that are essential for good health, a healthy reproductive system, and a better shot at becoming pregnant.

Zinc for your man

Zinc is an important mineral for everyone but especially for your male partner while you are trying to conceive. Zinc is found in high levels in the male reproductive parts and is necessary for proper reproductive functioning in men. Low levels of zinc in the diet can lead to both low testosterone levels and reduced sperm count and motility. The good news is that most men probably get plenty of zinc if they eat a healthy and well-balanced diet. The DRI for men 19 years and older is 11 mg daily. You can get plenty of zinc through foods such as extra-lean beef, poultry, seafood, oysters (very high in zinc), beans, oatmeal, fortified breakfast cereals, wheat germ, milk, nuts, and seeds.

Vitamin A

Any vitamin that contributes to the growth and health of body cells and tissues is going to get special attention during conception and pregnancy. And that includes vitamin A. In addition, this fat-soluble vitamin promotes normal vision, helps to regulate the immune system and works as an antioxidant in the form of carotenoids such as beta-carotene. Vitamin A is also important for the production of sperm, and we all know that when it comes to sperm, more is better! However, keep in mind that vitamin A is a different story for the ladies. As I mentioned earlier in the book, too much vitamin A (preformed) can be toxic for women during pregnancy. It isn't too hard to get what you need daily, especially if you are eating a healthy diet. Preformed vitamin A can be found in liver, milk, and fortified breakfast cereals and eggs, as well as in most supplements unless otherwise specified. Vitamin A in the form of beta-carotene can be found in orange, red, yellow, and dark green vegetables and fruits, such as carrots, cantaloupes, sweet potatoes, and spinach, just to name a few.

Vitamin C

Vitamin C is a water-soluble vitamin that is involved in many important functions in the body, and for the topic of trying to conceive, this vitamin acts as an antioxidant to help protect the interior and exterior of male sperm cells, helping to prevent sperm defects and boost motility. Eat plenty of foods rich in vitamin C such as citrus fruits, broccoli, potatoes with the skin, strawberries and other berries, kiwis, melons, peppers, tomatoes, kale, spinach, and cabbage. Note that your best sources of vitamin C are fruits and vegetables, so try to get your recommended servings in daily.

Vitamin E

Vitamin E is yet another vitamin that may help to increase sperm production and motility as well as help immature sperm to develop. This fat-soluble vitamin acts as a powerful antioxidant, which helps protect cells from damage—not only body cells but sperm cells, as well. You can find vitamin E in vegetable oils such as canola, flaxseed, olive, and sunflower oil. Fortified cereals and whole grains, sunflower seeds, almonds, avocados, spinach, and other greens are just a few more foods that are good sources of vitamin E.

Vitamin D

Vitamin D is a fat-soluble vitamin that is important to health and fertility. It promotes the absorption of calcium and phosphorus in the blood, regulates normal levels of these minerals, and helps to deposit them in the bones and teeth. Vitamin D also regulates cell growth and plays an important role in keeping our immune system healthy. When it comes to fertility, vitamin D is necessary to produce sex hormones, without the right balance of which you might suffer from problems such as PCOS, PMS, and infertility. Studies have shown that women with insufficient vitamin D levels have a higher risk of ovulation problems, which proves how important vitamin D is to the delicate reproductive system.

There are actually two ways to get vitamin D. One is through fortified foods such as milk, cereals (check the label), and certain brands of yogurt; fattier fish such as salmon, tuna, and mackerel; cod liver oil; and egg yolks, especially from fortified eggs. Some fortified egg brands can provide as much as 40 IU of vitamin D per egg compared to a regular or non-fortified egg, which provides about 21 IU's. Believe it or not, the other way we can get vitamin is through good old sunshine. Your body makes vitamin D when your skin is directly exposed to the sun. That doesn't mean you need to go out and spend hours in the sun, and given the risk of skin cancer, you shouldn't. Getting just10 to 15 minutes of exposure a day can be beneficial.

Recently the Institute of Medicine set new DRI's for Vitamin D. Not counting the vitamin D you get from sunshine, and assuming you are getting adequate amounts of calcium, they recommend an intake of 15 mcg (600 IU) daily for both men and women between the ages of 9 and 70 years. They advise not to get more then 100 mcg (4,000 IU) daily.

Vitamin B6

When trying to conceive there is a whole list of B vitamins that are important to properly nourish your body with, such as folic acid, vitamin B12, and vitamin B6. Vitamin B6 stands out as a nutrient that can give you a bit of an edge in the baby-making process. Vitamin B6 is important for a healthy immune system, enzyme function, protein metabolism, and production of red blood cells. As far as fertility is concerned, vitamin B6 helps to regulate hormones. Being deficient in this vitamin can cause irregular periods, progesterone imbalances, and poor egg quality, and on the men's side, poor sperm development. This B vitamin can also help to lengthen your *luteal phase*, or that time between ovulation and your menstrual period. You might know it as the "two- week wait." This time frame should last at least 11 to 16 days normally. If it is shorter than 10 days (which is considered too short to sustain a pregnancy), you could have a luteal phase defect. Vitamin B6 can also be helpful once you become pregnant by helping to alleviate the symptoms of morning sickness.

You may need a bit more then what is recommended daily (the DRI is 1.3 mg for women 19 to 50 years of age) to boost fertility and correct luteal defects, but keep in mind that too much can upset the balance of other essential B vitamins. Very high doses of supplemental B6 (500 to 1,000 mg per day) over a prolonged period of time can also result in neurological symptoms known as *sensory neuropathy*. Most women seem to have good results from just 50 mg per day of B6, which is a good place to start. Most women can take up to 200 mg per day safely. When taking B6 it is important to take a prenatal or multivitamin/mineral supplement that contains all of the B vitamins as they work together to get their jobs done and improve absorption into the body.

Vitamin B6 can be found in a wide variety of foods, including fortified cereals, poultry, beef, pork, fish, beans/legumes, and peanut butter, as well as some nuts, fruits, and vegetables. If you have questions about how much B6 you are taking or should be taking, and whether or not you may have a luteal phase defect, speak with your healthcare provider.

Special Precautions for Men

At any one second in time a man is creating thousands of new sperm, and that calls for an ample supply of micronutrients such as folic acid, iron, zinc, and all of the other ones I have mentioned so far. However, the same rules apply for men as for women. Don't overdo it on the vitamin and minerals. Mega doses do more harm than good. If you are taking any type of supplements for additional protein, to increase muscle mass, or for any other reason, check the label for additional vitamins and minerals that may be putting you over the top. Also be sure those supplements are not full of processed soy, as discussed in Chapter 4, or DHEA, a hormone-like substance that can cause fertility problems. Just as for women, if you are trying to conceive, speak with your healthcare provider about any supplements and medications you are taking.

Choosing A Prenatal Vitamin/Mineral Supplement

Most women who are actively trying to conceive can benefit from taking a prenatal supplement. You should at least be taking multivitamin/mineral supplement before trying to conceive and then consider switching to a prenatal once you begin actively trying to conceive. Even though you might be eating more healthily and taking better care of yourself, a prenatal can act as an insurance policy of sorts to cover any missing areas and to ensure you are getting the right amounts of essential nutrients during pregnancy. Just be careful not to rely on your supplement too heavily. It doesn't mean you can leave out certain food groups or take a step back from healthy eating. It is only meant to supplement a healthy diet, not take the place of food groups.

There are many prenatal supplements to choose from, but unfortunately the FDA doesn't regulate what goes into them, so no standards have been set as to what should be in them. A good prenatal supplement will provide at least the important nutrients we discussed previously, such as folic acid and iron, and shouldn't provide more then the recommended amounts of other nutrients, such a preformed vitamin A. Some prenatal supplements contain essential fatty acids (omega-3 fats) and some do not. Some contain more or less of essential nutrients and some contain herbs, as well. You can buy prenatals over the counter, or your healthcare provider can prescribe them. Your best bet is to make a preconception visit with your healthcare provider once you know you are ready to begin the conception journey and discuss with him/her which one will best fit your individual needs. Discuss with your healthcare provider any other supplements and/or medications you may be taking, and do not take additional supplements without talking to him/her first.

Some women have a problem with prenatals causing nausea. If this occurs, take it at night and make sure to take it with food. If it continues to bother you, talk to your healthcare provider about trying a different brand.

Powerhouse Fertility Foods

It may be time to begin a healthier way of eating, but that doesn't mean you need to feel deprived while you are trying to conceive. Healthy foods can be tasty and satisfying and can add that extra fertility boost you need. Of course no one food will boost fertility, but there are some foods that stick out as chock full of the nutrients most important to baby making. Eating these foods will not guarantee a pregnancy, but they are healthy foods that will ensure you are getting the nutrients you need. In addition, they will help boost your energy levels, prevent disease, and help you feel your best. You can't go wrong fueling your body with a combination of these nutritional powerhouse foods. This is only a limited list of nutrient-filled, fertility-friendly foods. There are many more out there to try, but this will get you started on the right path.

- **Broccoli:** This low-calorie vegetable is loaded with nutrients necessary for a healthy pregnancy as well as disease -fighting antioxidants such as vitamin A and C, beta-carotene, folate, calcium, and fiber. This isn't the only vegetable that is full of these essential nutrients. Be sure to eat a variety of vegetables each day. Try broccoli lightly streamed or raw and toss it with other veggies to rev up the nutrients and taste.

- **Bananas:** At just about 100 calories each, bananas are a good source of potassium, fiber, vitamin B6, and vitamin C. They can help increase your energy and add to your daily fruit intake. Some studies have found that couples who have lower than average intakes of foods high in antioxidants, such as fruits and veggies, had more fertility problems—so eat up! Mix bananas into smoothies, add them to your morning cereal, or eat one on the go or after a workout for a boost. As with veggies, eat a variety of fruits each day for maximum nutritional benefits.

- **Salmon:** Fish in general is loaded with healthy omega-3 fats though some are higher then others. Salmon is a fattier fish that is full of omega-3 fats and is one that is lower in mercury content. Eat a variety of fish but stick with the guidelines of the FDA and EPA.

- **Milk:** A diet rich in calcium is vital for strong bones and teeth, not to mention it can cut your risk for hypertension and certain cancers and help ease symptoms of PMS. Milk is a valuable source of calcium, vitamin D, vitamin A, riboflavin, niacin, and vitamin B12, all nutrients that are important to good fertility. Just one 8-ounce glass will supply close to one-third of your daily calcium requirements. If you are not a fan of milk, try making a smoothie out of it with fruit or use it on your favorite cereal. There are all kinds of ways to sneak milk into your diet; don't forget about other dairy foods such as yogurt and cheese.

- **Walnuts:** Nuts are a healthy food, probably much healthier then you realize. Most nuts and seeds are great sources of omega-3 fats, but walnuts in particular have one of the highest concentration. And let's not forget how important omega-3 fats are to productive baby-making and also a healthy baby. They are a good source of monounsaturated fats, as well, along with manganese and copper. Eating walnuts has many potential health benefits, ranging from heart health and improved cholesterol to better cognitive function and anti-inflammatory benefits. Walnuts contain high levels of L-arginine, an essential amino acid that helps improve the circulation to reproductive organs.

Walnuts, along with pecans and chestnuts, have some of the highest levels of antioxidants of all the tree nuts. Walnuts as well as other nuts and seeds are a delicious way to add a boost of nutrition, flavor, and crunch to any dish, including baked goods, soups, sauces, cooked vegetables, stuffing, stews, and salads. In addition, they make a convenient and highly nutritious snack. Just keep in mind that nuts and seeds are also full of calories, so watch your portion sizes.

- **Orange Juice/Oranges:** We have already read how important folate and vitamin C are to good health and fertility as well as to a healthy pregnancy. Look no further than your ordinary orange or a glass of orange juice to get a great source of both. Opt for the calcium-fortified orange juice and you can add another nutrient to the list. Citrus fruits are great sources of vitamin C, so keep plenty of them on hand.

- **Spinach:** There was a good reason your Mom always told you to eat your spinach. Dark green leafy vegetables such as spinach are packed with nutritional value, including folate, vitamin A, vitamin C, iron, and even calcium. Opt for darker greens in your salads to increase your nutritional intake. Try them on sandwiches or stir them into soup and pasta dishes.

- **Oatmeal:** Oatmeal is a whole grain and the perfect way to get a good healthy start to your day. Instead of choosing an instant oatmeal, which may be loaded with added sugar, cook up the plain type and add some sweetness of your own by adding cinnamon, raisins, or nuts for an added boost. Not a fan of oatmeal? Try a dry, whole-grain fortified cereal. Both will load you up on complex carbohydrates, fiber, and other essential nutrients essential for successful conception.

- **Peanut Butter:** No need to feel guilty snacking on a spoonful of peanut butter right from the jar. Peanut butter is loaded with good fertility stuff, including protein, potassium, magnesium, calcium, niacin, fiber, iron, zinc, and vitamin E. Yes, it contains fat, but luckily it is the "good" fat, or unsaturated type of fat. Peanut butter on a piece of whole-wheat bread can make the perfect combination for breakfast, lunch, or a quick snack. As do all nuts, peanut butter can pack in the calories, so watch your serving sizes.

- **Sweet Potatoes:** These are the spuds to choose! They should be a staple in your diet and not just show up at the holiday dinner table. Sweet potatoes are an excellent source of potassium, fiber, vitamin C, and beta-carotene, a powerful antioxidant.

- **Whole-Grain Bread:** One simple change of swapping white bread for whole-grain bread can do wonders for your nutritional intake. Whole grain breads offer so much more including protein, fiber, iron, zinc, and plenty of B vitamins. Don't forget about the switch to other whole grains found in whole-grain pasta, brown rice, and whole-grain cereals. Keep in mind that whole grains have less of an effect on blood sugar and insulin as compared to refined grains (white bread, white rice, and white pasta). Anything that affects insulin less is good for fertility.

- **Eggs:** Eggs are versatile and another great way to get high-quality protein. They are also full of riboflavin, vitamin B12, and vitamin D. Eggs also contribute choline to our diets. A choline deficiency can actually cause a deficiency of folic acid. Eggs can be a great alternative to meat for those who are not meat eaters and for those many pregnant women who develop an aversion to meat. Add some chopped-up vegetables to your eggs for a healthy breakfast, lunch, or dinner and you have a complete meal. Egg yolks can also be high in cholesterol, so eat them in moderation.

- **Tomatoes:** This vegetable (actually it's a fruit) is loaded with a long list of vitamins, minerals, antioxidants, and phytonutrients. Most importantly, tomatoes provide lycopene, which is a powerful disease-fighting antioxidant and just possibly may be an added fertility booster. Add tomatoes to all sorts of salads, casseroles, pasta dishes, soups, and stews. They make a great snack, too!

- **Dried Beans and Legumes:** A fertility-friendly diet should include some protein from plant sources. Dried beans, legumes, and lentils are all excellent low-fat sources of protein. They are also good sources of iron, fiber, folate, zinc, and potassium. They are also delicious, inexpensive, and versatile. Popular varieties include pinto beans, kidney beans, black beans, navy beans, lentils, split peas, and chickpeas. They are great in salads, soups, casseroles, pasta dishes, rice dishes, and stews. Try a non-meat meal a few times a week and use beans as the perfect substitution.

This list of foods will give you a good place to start and give you an idea of just how nutritious healthy foods can be. Be brave and branch out to try all types of healthy foods. The more variety you eat, the greater the nutritional benefit for good reproductive health and that fertility edge.

Chapter 6

Fertility-Friendly Alternative Therapies

Treatments to boost fertility are plentiful. They range from concepts we have already discussed, such as lifestyle and diet, to medical procedures to alternative therapies. Many couples opt for a combination of treatments to help increase their chances of conception. The types of treatments we will talk about in this chapter are alternative therapies.

Alternative therapies—or, more specifically, complimentary and alternative medicine (CAM)—can be defined in many ways. For our purposes we will define them as any healing practices that don't fall under the umbrella of conventional medicine. CAM isn't for everyone and it should be a choice you make along with your healthcare provider. This chapter will discuss some of the alternative treatments that are most popular with couples trying to conceive, along with some of the pros, cons, and safety concerns that go along with them.

The Scoop on Herbs

It is quite common for couples to want to try natural or alternative ways to boost their fertility, and many times herbs top the list. There is no question that the verdict is still out for many scientific and health experts on the use of dietary supplements in the form of herbs for increasing your chances of trying to conceive. On one hand, herbs have traditionally been used for all types of physical and mental health issues—including fertility—for centuries in many parts of the world. In fact, experts such as herbalists, naturopaths, and some acupuncturists who specialize in fertility can be very knowledgeable about the use, effectiveness, and safety of herbs and herbal blends. On the flip side, many conventional medical doctors and other healthcare professionals may not recommend them and feel that even though research is ongoing, there is not yet enough definitive research to prove their effectiveness and safety.

The use of herbs should be taken just as seriously as the use of prescription and over-the-counter medications. They work much in the same way as conventional drugs through naturally occurring chemical reactions in the body. Even though herbs are natural, "natural" doesn't necessarily mean that they are guaranteed safe and effective. Just as with any other medication, they can have potential side effects and drug interactions. In fact, it is a good idea to be even more cautious with these products because even though the FDA regulates dietary supplements such as herbs, the regulations are much less strict then those for prescription medications and over-the-counter drugs. Always seek professional advice before using any type of herb or herbal blend. Even herbs that are deemed safe may not be appropriate for everyone.

FYI: Herbal supplements are classified as a type of dietarary supplement and can contain a single herb or a mixture of herbs. An herb is defined as a plant or plant part (such as flowers, seeds, or leaves) that is used for its flavor, scent, and/or therapeutic properties. The word "botanical" is often used in place of the word "herb."

Points to keep in mind concerning the use of herbs:

- Gather information about the herb you are considering using from reputable sources such as the ones listed in Chapter 9. Do not rely on information that is being provided by the manufacturer or the seller of the product.

- Keep in mind that some herbs can interact with medications or other dietary supplements you may be taking and can contain ingredients that are not listed on the label. This can be especially true if you are already taking prescription medications for fertility treatments.

- Federal regulations for dietary supplements such as herbs are very different from those for other medications. For instance, manufacturers of dietary supplements do not have to prove a product's safety and effectiveness before it is put on the market. In addition, the manufacturer's use of the terms "standardized," "verified," or "certified" do not guarantee a product's consistency, purity, or quality. What is on the label may not always be what is in the bottle.

- When taking an herbal supplement, read and follow the label instructions. Stop the supplement and contact your healthcare provider if you experience any side effects.

- Don't expect herbal supplements to be a quick fix. Many of them take months or more of use before they become effective, if they ever do.

- Don't rely on herbal supplements as your only method of boosting fertility. You need to first start with the basics of making positive lifestyle changes with diet, vitamin/mineral intake, and exercise as well as other habits. Don't use herbs as a magic cure and/or your only means of boosting fertility.

- Always, always, always discuss your use of herbs and other dietary supplements with your healthcare provider and let them know about all medications you are taking. Talk to them about a dosage that is safe and effective for your situation.

- Keep in mind that if you are taking an herbal supplement to help you conceive, you could become pregnant while taking the supplement, so be sure it is safe during pregnancy or that you stop the supplement in plenty of time to get it out of your system before pregnancy can occur.

• Never misuse dietary supplements as they can be just as dangerous as the misuse of any other medication and can work to decrease your fertility instead of increasing it.

Herbs for Fertility

Countless herbs are touted as being able to improve the repro-ductive process and therefore increase fertility. Many herbs come as blends, with several herbs combined in one supplement. The premise is that they have a synergistic effect when used in combination with each other that is greater than the effects of the individual herbs. Just as there are numerous herbs that are believed to increase fertility, such as red clover, partridge berry, liferoot, wild carrot, and wild yam, there are just as many that should be avoided, as they can have a negative impact on the baby-making process. Some studies have found that herbs such as St. John's wort, echinacea, and ginkgo biloba can be harmful to sperm. Others, such as black cohosh, chasteberry, ephedra, fennel, flaxseed, ginseng, goldenseal juniper, lavender, licorice root, St. John's wort, and thyme, are said to be hazardous if used during the luteal phase (after ovulation) of the menstrual cycle and/or during pregnancy, even though some of these are used to enhance fertility if used with the right timing. This is only a short list of what you should not take after ovulation or during pregnancy. Be sure you know the facts about any herbal supple-ment before you take it.

Herbs come in a variety of forms, including whole herbs that are dried and developed into a powdered form for use; teas, either lose or in a tea bag; capsules and tablets; and extracts, which usually offer higher concentrations. For just about all herbs and herbal supplements, proven scientific evidence that they do what they say they do is still very scarce, so keep that in mind as you read through the information, and don't be afraid to do some of your own research. Just because an herb is touted as having certain properties or abilities or because it is used for certain issues doesn't necessarily mean that it is guaranteed to help or scientifi-cally proven to do what it claims. The following are just a few of the most popular herbs that are used for fertility and the claims they may make.

Black Cohosh

This herb has been used for evening out menstrual irregularities, reducing PMS symptoms, and increasing fertility. In addition, it has been used to induce labor in pregnant women by stimulating the uterus, so it is important not to use this herb if you become pregnant as it may initiate a miscarriage if taken in too high a dose. Only take this herb after speaking to an expert regarding dosage and the safest time to take it during your cycle. Do not take this herb while breastfeeding. Study results are mixed on whether black cohosh is effective or not.

False Unicorn Root

This herb has long been used to encourage fertility in women and treat impotence in men. False unicorn root contains hormone-like substances that are believed to help balance sex hormones and relieve disorders of the reproductive tract, menstrual irregularities, and PMS. It has been used to help normalize the ovaries and improve egg formation within the ovaries. Taking too much of this herb may cause health issues such as hot flashes, stomach and kidney issues, and possible blurred vision, so take only recommended doses.

Wild Yam

This herb contains a plant estrogen that seems to be a precursor to progesterone, which helps to increase the production of this hormone in the body. An increase in progesterone can aid with short luteal phases or a luteal phase defect. This herb should be taken after ovulation because if taken before, it may actually prevent ovulation.

Red Clover

This herb is thought to help heal scarring of the fallopian tubes, regulate menstrual cycles, eliminate abnormal cells in the reproductive tract, and minister to "unexplained" infertility. Red clover is quite nourishing in that it contains plenty of vitamins, as well as minerals such as calcium, magnesium, selenium, and zinc. It is said to be useful in helping to balance hormones and support the reproductive organs, all contributing to better fertility health. Scientific testing has also found high levels of *isoflavone*, which is a plant-based chemical that has estrogen-like effects in the body, much like soy. In addition, red clover supposedly has an alkalinizing effect on the entire body, which may help to create a more sperm-friendly environment. This herb, like most others, is still being studied to learn more about its active components and effectiveness. Because red clover contains estrogen-like compounds, it is unclear whether it is safe for women who are pregnant, breastfeeding, or who have hormone-sensitive cancers such as breast cancer, so it is best to err on the side of caution.

Wheatgrass

Wheatgrass tends to be a popular supplement for women trying to conceive. It is a nutrient-rich type of young grass that is in the wheat family. It is often sold in a variety of forms as a dietary supplement. Proponents say that extracting the juice is the best way to reap its benefits, though you can also find it in tablet, capsule, and tincture form. Wheatgrass in its juice form can have a strong grassy taste, making it difficult to swallow. Wheatgrass provides a high concentration of nutrients including iron, calcium, magnesium, certain amino acids, and chlorophyll, as well as vitamins A, C, and E. This supplement has been in the spotlight for its "curative powers," and there is talk that it can boost fertility, though it isn't quite clear yet which components of wheatgrass do the boosting. However, as we know there are no magic cures, and studies are not strong enough to show evidence of these fertility-boosting powers. Wheatgrass is generally considered safe but can cause side effects in some people, such as nausea, headaches, hives, or swelling of the throat. It is advised not to use wheatgrass if you are pregnant or breastfeeding or if you are allergic to wheat, have celiac disease, or gluten intolerance.

Chasteberry

Chasteberry, or *vitex*, is another popular herb used to increase fertility and ease PMS symptoms. This herb is said to stimulate the pituitary gland, which is responsible for producing and balancing hormones such as estrogen, progesterone, and testosterone. This in turn may help regulate menstrual cycles and/or lengthen the luteal phase, both of which can increase your chances of conceiving. Studies are ongoing with this herb and there doesn't seem to be enough reliable scientific evidence at this point to determine whether chasteberry is effective in increasing fertility, although evidence does support using it to relieve symptoms of PMS. Chasteberry is normally well-tolerated but has been associated with some side effects such as dizziness, headaches, dry mouth, skin rashes, and gastrointestinal symptoms. Because this herb may affect certain hormone levels, it is advised that women who are pregnant or who have hormone-sensitive conditions such as breast cancer avoid its use. Certain medications should also not be used with this herb, so check with your healthcare provider before using it.

Dong Quai

Don Quai is an herb that has been used for centuries to help solve menstrual irregularities and balance estrogen levels in the body. This herb works by promoting blood flow to the pelvis region to help circulation and also to strengthen and balance the uterus improving the chances for implantation. Don Quai is said to have a relaxing effect on the uterus, which may also be helpful for PMS symptoms and cramping during the menstrual cycle. Although Don Quai is considered safe for most people, there are some who should not use it, including pregnant women, women who are breastfeeding, people with bleeding disorders, women with excessive menstrual bleeding, people who are experiencing diarrhea and/or the flu, women with breast cancer, and people taking blood thinners.

Evening Primrose Oil

Evening primrose oil has been used for years for skin conditions and rheumatoid arthritis but more recently is being used for women's health issues such as breast pain associated with the menstrual cycle, menopausal symptoms, and PMS. In addition, it is used to improve the quality and fertility of cervical mucus, which is helpful in pinpointing ovulation and necessary to nourish, protect, and speed sperm on their way to fertilize the egg. Evening primrose oil is rich in vitamin E as well as an essential fatty acid called gamma linolenic acid (GLA). This herb is usually well-tolerated by most people with only mild side effects such as headache. Scientific evidence is not strong that it lives up to the hype, however.

Green Tea

Green tea seems to be a popular addition to many women's daily routine when they are trying to conceive. There is no harm in drinking a cup or two a day while you are baby making, but don't expect it to significantly increase your odds. Although green tea is full of antioxidants and other compounds that offer some protective health benefits, research hasn't been quite as positive for boosting fertility. If you do decide to drink green tea, you may want to opt for the caffeine free varieties, as too much caffeine has been linked to fertility problems. Green tea has much less caffeine than coffee and other teas, but if you trying to cut it out keep in mind that your green tea may include it.

Other Dietary Supplements

There are a few other types of dietary supplements, aside from herbs, that are touted as having fertility-boosting properties.

L-Arginine

L-arginine is an amino acid needed to make protein in the body. It is considered only semi-essential because our body can make it under normal conditions. We can also get it from protein foods in our diets, including red meat, poultry, fish, dairy products, and some nuts. In addition, you can find it in synthetic form in supplements. L-arginine is used for various health conditions including heart and blood vessel conditions, chest pain, high blood pressure, coronary artery disease, dementia, erectile dysfunction, female sexual problems, and male infertility. Some people use L-arginine in supplement form to improve athletic performance and boost the immune system; however, the amino acid has not been proven to be effective for either. L-arginine is often used in combination with both over-the-counter and/or prescription medications for a variety of conditions.

L-arginine works by being converted in the body into a chemical called nitric oxide. Nitric oxide in turn helps the blood vessels open up for better blood flow. This increased blood flow is what is believed to help improve circulation to the reproductive organs in both males and females, thus boosting fertility. Nitric oxide may help increase sperm count and sperm motility in men, and increase cervical mucus in women. L-arginine also may stimulate certain hormones in the body, such as insulin, growth hormone (GH), and glucagon. It is not certain how safe L-arginine is during pregnancy and breastfeeding, so it is best to avoid it during these times. Though the L-arginine we consume through foods is safe, taken in higher doses through supplements may cause some side effects, including diarrhea, stomach problems, and low blood pressure. If you are interested in this supplement, speak with your healthcare provider concerning a dosage that is right for you. At this time there seems to be insufficient evidence to rate the effectiveness for both male infertility and female sexual problems.

L-Carnitine

L-carnitine is another amino acid used to build protein in the body. This is another amino acid that is only semi-essential because our body is able to produce what we need daily, and we can acquire it from some of the foods that we eat. L-carnitine occurs in two forms, but it is L-carnitine that is active in the body and is the type you find naturally in foods. You can find L-carnitine mostly in red meats, fish, poultry, and dairy products. Even though we make what we need daily, there are synthetic forms that are used in supplements. L-carnitine, acetyl-L-carnitine, and propionyl-L-carnitine are all forms used in over-the-counter dietary supplements, which are promoted for use in a number of situations.

One important function of L-carnitine in the body is its critical role in energy production. In addition, L-carnitine is essential for normal function of sperm cells, including sperm formation and maturation.

According to research, it appears that the higher the level of L-carnitine in the sperm cell, the better the sperm count and motility. More studies are needed to add evidence that supplementing with additional L-carnitine has potential value as an infertility therapy. As always, speak with your healthcare provider concerning the use and dosage of this amino acid before taking it. Some side effects can occur, including nausea, vomiting, diarrhea, and abdominal cramping.

Flaxseed and Flaxseed Oil

Some may call flaxseed one of the most powerful plant foods around. Flaxseed and its derivative, flaxseed oil, are rich in an abundance of healthy components, including the essential fatty acid ALA, which we know from a previous chapter is a precursor to the healthy omega-3 fatty acids. Actual flaxseeds are also rich in B vitamins, magnesium, and manganese as well as plant estrogens known as *lignans*, which also boast antioxidant properties. Flaxseeds contain lignans whereas the oil of flaxseeds does not. Some experts say that flaxseeds are a powerful package that can help balance hormones, improve uterine function, and boost female fertility. Flaxseed is often used to treat symptoms of PMS as well as menopause. Your best choice when it comes to flaxseed is to opt for ground flaxseeds that you can sprinkle over oatmeal, yogurt, soups, or salads or blend into a smoothie. Flaxseed contains plenty of both soluble and insoluble fiber so it may have a laxative effect for some. If you decide to add flaxseed to your diet, treat it as you would a fiber supplement and introduce it slowly into your diet and drink plenty of water. Experts generally recommend one to two tablespoons of ground flaxseed per day as a suggested dose for good health.

Flaxseed oil is said to play a role in promoting male fertility. It is believed that the components of flaxseed oil help keep sperm healthy. Some experts believe this holds true for women, as well, and that adding flaxseed oil to your daily diet may be a simple way to give your fertility a bit of a boost. Flaxseed oil can have an odd taste, so many people take the oil in the form of a supplement capsule. Keep in mind that flaxseed oil is only part of the flaxseed and thus doesn't contain all of the same components.

> *FYI: Ground flaxseed is more digestible then whole flax-seed. You can buy flaxseed whole and grind it yourself or buy it already ground. Ground flaxseed doesn't keep very long so your best bet is to store it in the freezer. Don't be confused by different product names: "milled," "ground" and "flax meal" all mean the same thing.*

The effects of flaxseeds and flaxseed oil on fertility are not exactly well-established; however, they seem to be safe for most people. With all of the healthy components they possess, they most definitely can't hurt. Keep in mind, though, that because of the plant estrogens they contain, some warn against using whole or ground flaxseed during pregnancy and breastfeeding. It is best to err on the side of caution and speak to your healthcare provider if you are using or are planning on using flaxseeds and/or flaxseed oil.

Don't Let Stress Get to You

For some of us it is easier said than done! But letting go of everyday stress might just boost your chances of conceiving. Stress may not be the actual cause of infertility, but the effect that it has on the body, such as causing hormonal imbalances or lowering sperm count, can add to fertility problems. Hormonal imbalances can cause you to ovulate later in your cycle or cause menstrual irregularities, making it more difficult to become pregnant. In fact, some studies show that more couples get pregnant during months that they reported feeling happy and relaxed, as opposed to months when they were stressed, anxious, or worried.

Stress might not have anything to do with diet, but trying to conceive requires a complete package, so if you are eating right but not taking care of yourself in other ways you might be putting up a roadblock to success. If trying to conceive stresses you out this can lead to a vicious cycle of "you can't conceive so you get stressed, and the stress keeps you from conceiving." And this doesn't only pertain to women!

Stress can cause fertility problems for men, too. But don't let the thought of stress, stress you out even more! There are techniques you can use to help manage your stress, and that includes stress you may have about trying to conceive, the stress that piles up on a daily basis, and stress that can come from traumatic life events. Everyone handles stress differently, but if you know you have a hard time managing stress, it is time to do something about it.

We already discussed one form of stress relief earlier in the book, and that was exercise. A regular exercise routine can help you reduce stress. In addition, eating a healthy diet, meditating, using other alternative therapies, getting adequate sleep, journal writing, massage, and talking to friends and family can help reduce everyday stress. What is an effective stress-relieving technique for one person may not work for another. Find what works for you!

Using Alternative Therapies

Recent research has found that alternative therapies are becoming much more common among those who are trying to learn how to reduce stress and boost their chances of becoming pregnant. There are many types of alternative therapies to try, but the key is finding one that you feel comfortable with and is a good fit. Keep in mind that none of these therapies should be your ultimate answer to conception. There can be complex and numerous issues that contribute to a couple's infertility. It is the whole package that will be most beneficial, so make sure that the alternative therapies you choose are coupled with a healthy diet, regular exercise, a healthy lifestyle, and good overall health.

Motivation to try alternative therapies can also be a cost issue for those having problems becoming pregnant as they can cost much less then medical therapy such as in-vitro fertilization. Many couple may even compliment their medical therapies with alternative therapies to increase their chances even more. There are no guarantees but they can't hurt if you are game to try them. Not to mention they can swing some positive energy in your direction and who can't use that.

? *What is yoga and can it help?*

While practicing the ancient discipline of yoga isn't a one-way ticket to successfully becoming pregnant, it can help reduce your stress levels and therefore boost your chances. Yoga is holistic, meaning it combines both mind and body.

Yoga can have a very calming effect depending on the type you choose. Opt for yoga that is conducive to fertility issues and includes a gentle, meditating, and relaxing style over one that is more vigorous. Yoga that is specific to fertility is meant to stimulate and tone the reproductive system, improve the flow of energy and circulation through the body, balance hormone levels, and provide relaxation. You might even bring your male partner along and practice yoga together as it can benefit both of you. It is very important for anyone who wants to become pregnant and/or is having fertility issues to have a complete physical before beginning yoga practice. Seek out yoga instructors who specialize in fertility, if possible. The great news is that once you do become pregnant you can continue with your yoga, which can help to relieve tension and strengthen your body in preparation for birth. But again, make sure you work with an instructor who specializes in pregnancy yoga and receive clearance from your healthcare provider first.

? *What is Reiki and can it help?*

With the rise in popularity of Reiki therapy, you may be thinking it is something new but it is far from that. Reiki is an ancient form of natural Japanese healing that has been around for many centuries. The term *reiki* actually means "spiritually guided life energy" or, more commonly, "universal life energy." Treatments are based on the channeling and balancing of positive energy within the body, through a practitioner, to promote overall health and healing. Reiki therapy sends the body into a deep state of relaxation, which is said to unlock the body's own healing powers. This therapy is meant to address physical, emotional, mental, and spiritual imbalances. There are a variety of benefits that are said to be associated with Reiki treatments including reduced stress and anxiety levels, increased energy levels, improved the immune system, reduced muscle pain, and improved fertility.

There isn't much you have to do during a Reiki treatment except to be open to the process. During the session, the practitioner uses gentle hand movements to channel positive energy from his/her hands into the patient. Hand movements hover just above the patient's body and are often performed without body contact, depending on whether other therapies are being used in conjunction with Reiki. When you receive a Reiki treatment specifically for trying to conceive, the practitioner will focus on balancing the energy in certain areas of your body (mainly the reproductive region) called *chakras*. Chakras are energy centers within the body where it is believed that energy enters and leaves the body and also where healing energies can get stuck or clogged. Reiki energy needs to be able to flow freely throughout the body. If it can't, the regions located in the area of the energy block can cease to function properly. A Reiki treatment is probably one of the most relaxing treatments you will ever experience and one worth a try.

Because the purpose of Reiki is to improve overall physical and mental health, it can in turn improve your chances of conceiving by promoting better overall health, including reproductive health. In addition, it may help minimize conditions and illnesses that may be contributing to infertility. Just as with other forms of alternative therapy, Reiki can be beneficial for both men and women and should be used in conjunction with other healthy lifestyle changes. Reiki therapy can also be beneficial during pregnancy to help reduce stress, improve sleep quality, and minimize morning sickness. Seek a Reiki therapist who is properly trained and qualified by inquiring about schooling, qualifications, and training.

? What is acupuncture and can it help?

Acupuncture is an ancient Chinese technique used to eliminate pain, relieve stress, and heal ailments. It is one of the most studied CAM therapies. Acupuncture is based on the belief that the human body's vital energy, or *chi*, flows along certain pathways in the body and needs to be in balance for the body to be healthy and function properly. Depending on the ailment, different sizes of thin, sharp needles are gently inserted into specific acupuncture points on the body to stimulate and rebalance the body's energy in those areas. This is meant to release special hormones that trigger the natural healing process to let the body properly do its work. In addition, acupuncture is said to help regulate blood flow and release endorphins, which in turn can help relieve pain. Traditional acupuncture therapy is believed to treat the body as a whole as it regulates one's emotional, mental, spiritual, and physical balance. Even though the thought of needles may make you cringe, it is quite painless with few side effects, if any.

The verdict is still out on whether acupuncture can improve fertility or not. Some research suggests that its effectiveness in reducing stress can theoretically improve your odds of getting pregnant. Others believe that using this therapy to help increase blood flow to the uterus and surrounding areas and/or balance the hormones can also increase fertility odds. In addition, acupuncture is often recommended for use in conjunction with medical therapies such as IVF (in-vitro fertilization). Acupuncture is more of a process-oriented type of therapy, as are most CAM therapies, and you need to start before the fact and continue on a regular basis to hope for any type of therapeutic effect. There are not many risks when it comes to using acupuncture as a way to boost fertility. However, once you become pregnant, using incorrect pressure points can be risky, so it is always best to be treated by a properly trained and licensed acupuncturist specializing in fertility. Acupuncture itself is safe regardless of a person's health and/or medications; however, it is often is used in combination with herbal therapies, which can be contraindicated for certain health issues and medications. In most states acupuncture is a licensed profession, and therapists must be board certi-fied, so do your homework before you choose one to visit.

Acupuncture is most definitely not just for women who are trying to conceive. It has been found that men can benefit from it, as well. A few studies have shown that regular treatments may improve sperm count and motility as well as decrease the number of abnormal sperm.

Chapter 7

Navigating Unproven Diet Remedies

If you are actively trying to conceive, there is no doubt that you have read on the Internet or heard from a friend that eating enough of a specific food or group of foods will naturally help you conceive. Believe it or not, you can even find (non-scientifically based, of course) foods that will supposedly help you conceive the gender you are hoping for. Although it is tempting to believe there are specific conception-boosting foods out there, you can't believe everything you hear or read. Getting stuck on one or two foods that you believe can help you get pregnant can keep you from considering your diet as a whole and can also leave less room for a variety of healthy foods that will better balance your diet and boost your fertility. It might not hurt to add certain foods to your diet regimen, but just be sure you are balancing your dietary intake and not going overboard with any one food. The following is just a sampling of the most popular food remedies that have yet to be scientifically proven; there are plenty more where these came from.

Full-Fat Dairy Products Will Increase Fertility

The controversy in this strategy is whether full-fat is better for fertility then the fat-free and low-fat versions that are normally recommended for good health. Some studies have found that women eating as little as one serving of whole milk or other full-fat dairy product daily were less likely to experience infertility due to ovulatory issues. There is speculation that fat-free and low-fat dairy products contain an imbalance of sex hormones that could possibly affect ovulation and therefore conception. This is most certainly not a dietary change you would want to stick with long-term, as these foods are quite high in the "bad" saturated fats, which can be harmful to your health and your heart. This dietary recommendation is not based on solid science, but if you decide to try it, keep in mind what a single serving is and don't go overboard. If you have problems with cholesterol and/or have any type of heart problem, speak with your healthcare provider before making this type of dietary change.

Pineapple Will Increase the Chances of Implantation

The philosophy behind eating pineapple is that it contains an enzyme, called *bromelain*, which may be helpful for implantation of a fertilized egg because it helps to reduce inflammation within the uterus. The rule of thumb is that it must be fresh pineapple, as cooking and canning will destroy the components that supposedly help. The highest concentration of bromelain is found mostly in the core of the pineapple. It does have other health benefits, for example such as an anti-inflammatory and digestive aid. Because potential benefits probably come from more pineapple than one could consume in a regular meal, bromelain supplements have popped up on the market. There is no scientific research to prove bromelain's or pineapple's effectiveness for implantation. As a word of caution, eating too much pineapple too early in your cycle may create a more acidic cervical mucus, which is not ideal for sperm and conception. Pineapple, as with all fruit, is quite healthy, and even if it doesn't do what it is touted to do, it does contain plenty of disease-fighting antioxidants that can help strengthen the immune system. Your best bet is to eat it in moderation along with a variety of other fruits for good health.

Oysters Will Increase a Man's Fertility

You may have heard of the aphrodisiac effect oysters have, and obviously that can be helpful for conception. But there is some evidence that they can also improve sperm quality. The biggest scientific reasoning for this is that oysters contain high levels of zinc, which is needed to produce healthy sperm and promote sperm motility. Oysters are not the only way to get enough zinc in your man's diet, but they do provide a healthy dose compared to other foods.

Grapefruit Will Produce Better Cervical Mucus

Although there is no medical evidence to suggest drinking grapefruit juice will increase one's fertility, many women will swear that it helps to thin the cervical mucus, creating a more fertile environment for sperm and fertilization. To follow this remedy you need to drink grapefruit juice regularly for a couple of cycles before you begin to see any type of significant change. Even if the grapefruit juice doesn't work its magic on your cervical mucus, you can't go wrong with drinking fruit juice, as long as it 100-percent juice and doesn't contain added sugars. It will help to increase your fluids and add loads of essential nutrients to your daily diet. Keep in mind that there are medications out there that should *not* be taken with grapefruit, so check with your healthcare provider and/or local pharmacist if you take prescription medications before starting a regimen of grapefruit juice. If you drink grapefruit juice daily, remember to combine it with a variety of other whole fruits to make sure you are getting your daily number of servings of fruit and your fill of fiber.

Baby Carrots Will Increase Fertility

If you like baby carrots you may be in luck. The premise with this idea is that eating plenty of baby carrots may help produce more cervical mucus, which can give you a better chance at getting pregnant. Baby carrots are apparently very alkaline, which often helps unfriendly cervical mucus to become more accommodating to incoming sperm. Baby carrots are often used in conjunction with other simple remedies, such as drinking plenty of water and taking evening primrose oil, both of which supposedly create better cervical mucus, as well. Baby carrots are good for you and contain loads of essential nutrients, including fiber and vitamin A in the form of beta-carotene, a powerful antioxidant. There is not a whole lot of scientific data to back up this claim about baby carrots, but if you add them to your diet the worse thing that might happen is that you begin snacking on something healthy during the day and add more vegetables to your daily intake. The best thing that might happen is that it helps you to produce more sperm-friendly cervical mucus to aid in conception. Be careful not to choose carrots as your only vegetable throughout the day and as always don't go overboard. Keep in mind that it is important to consume a variety of vegetables each day to increase your nutrient intake, which is also beneficial to successful conception.

Bananas Will Increase a Man's Fertility

Bananas contain high levels of magnesium in addition to vitamin B6, vitamin C, potassium, and fiber. According to a small number of experts, eating bananas regularly can mean an increase in sperm count and a better chance at conceiving. Eating other foods high in magnesium may also have similar effects, assuming men avoid things such as alcohol, smoking, and hot showers or saunas, al of which can negatively affect sperm production. Although the scientific evidence on this one is a bit spotty, adding fruit to your daily diet never hurts.

Shitake Mushrooms Improve Sperm Health

Shitake mushrooms are very high in a strong antioxidant called L-ergothionein. Research has found that these mushrooms have much more of this antioxidant than the two foods that were always thought to contain the most: wheat germ and chicken liver. In addition, shitake mushrooms are an excellent source of selenium and a very good source of iron. They are also good sources of vitamin C, protein, and fiber. Because antioxidants can counteract seminal oxidative stress, which is known to have a significant negative effect on male fertility, eating these mushrooms is said to go a long way in improving sperm health and therefore increasing the chances of conception. Oysters, along with a few other types of mushrooms, also contribute high amounts of L-ergothioneine. If you are ready to add shitake mushrooms to your diet on a regular basis, be forewarned that they also contain high levels of purines. Some individuals are susceptible to purine-related problems, in which case excessive intake can cause health problems. Purines are broken down into uric acid, and health conditions such as gout and kidney stones are two examples of uric acid–related problems that can be linked to excessive intake of foods with purine. Know your health history before adding foods such as these and always stick to eating any food in moderation.

Molasses Can Help Increase Fertility

Molasses, specifically blackstrap molasses, seems to be a great natural supplement for women. It is very nutrient rich and is considered a sweetener that is actually good for you. It is said to help with PCOS, irregular periods, hormonal imbalances, and fatigue. Best-known are its affects on uterine fibroids, which can be detrimental to fertility by preventing the sperm from reaching the egg for fertilization. Blackstrap molasses contains calcium, iodine, iron, and other trace minerals that help to alkalinize the body and possibly discourage fibroid growth and shrink existing ones. In addition, its components are said to help decrease the chances of miscarriage. If this is something you wish to try, you can use blackstrap molasses as a substitute when baking, as an addition to baked beans, as a marinade for chicken or turkey, as a substitute for jelly on toast, or anywhere you would typically add something sweet.

Black Sesame Seeds Help Put Fertility in Top Shape

According to traditional Chinese medicine, black sesame seeds can enhance your liver "essence," or energy. According to Chinese medicine, when your liver is in top shape, so is your fertility and therefore your chances for conception. Black sesame seeds can usually be found at health food stores. They can be consumed alone, added to salads, or used in baking. You can also add them to your favorite bread topping and used on top of whole-wheat toast. As always, do not eat them in excess, as too much of any one food can throw off the very balance you are trying to achieve.

Chilies Can Increase Your Chances of Conception

If you like your food a little spicy you just might be in luck. Spicy foods containing red chili pepper apparently increase blood circulation throughout the body and provide a healthy blood supply to the reproductive area. In addition, chilies stimulate endorphin production, the feel-good hormone that is associated with stress release, which may help create a feeling of relaxation and increase your chances of conception. One more little tidbit: chilies are an excellent source of vitamin C, which can help greatly with iron absorption.

Garlic Helps Boost Nutrients Essential for Conception

Garlic breath isn't exactly known for its boost in romance, but garlic does contain an abundance of fertility-boosting nutrients. Garlic contains selenium, a mineral that is said to enhance male fertility and possibly reduce the chances of miscarriage in women. In addition, garlic contains vitamin B6, a vitamin needed to regulate hormones and strengthen the immune system. A deficiency in selenium and/or vitamin B6 is often implicated in fertility problems. So don't overlook the garlic. Even though it may not be fully proven it might just give you an extra fertility edge and give your favorite dishes and marinades a kick of flavor.

Honey Helps Boost Fertility

Not only is honey a great way to naturally sweeten your foods and beverages, but it has been used for centuries to help boost fertility. In fact, many deem honey to be a type of fertility-boosting superfood for both women and men. Honey is rich in minerals and amino acids (the building blocks of protein) that are central to good reproductive health, the stimulation of ovarian function, and the quality and quantity of sperm.

Chapter 8

Help Boost Your Chances With Delicious Recipes and Meal Plans

Reading about all the foods you should or should not include is one thing but transitioning them into your real life is another thing altogether. Life can get busy and hectic as we all know, and putting such recommendations into practice takes some thinking ahead and definite planning. To help give you a head start, I have included a variety of delicious recipes from other nutritional professionals that can add nutritional value and great flavor to your daily meal plans. Following easy recipes can teach you how to prepare tasty dishes that can make eating healthily taste good. Hopefully this will motivate you to take it a step further and experiment with other nutritious recipes from books, friends and family, and the Web, or even create your own tasty recipes. I have also included a week's worth of menu plans that will give you some ideas for putting the recommendations you have read about here into practice. Let them be a starting point to better managing your diet to help boost your fertility. For those trying to conceive, now is a better time than any to learn how to enjoy healthy foods every day. Bon appetit!

Main Entrees

Quick Lasagna
Makes 12 servings

3 cups low-fat cottage cheese or low-fat Ricotta cheese
2 Tbs. dried parsley
1 tsp. chopped garlic
4 cups spaghetti sauce (less than 4 grams fat per 4 ounces)*
3/4 pound uncooked lasagna noodles (12 noodles)
1 cup (4 oz.) grated, reduced-fat mozzarella cheese
1/4 cup grated Parmesan cheese

You don't precook the noodles in this recipe, so it is really fast to assemble. This can be put together the night before and refrigerated without baking.

Preheat oven to 350 degrees. Spray a 9 × 13-inch baking pan with nonstick cooking spray.

Mix cottage cheese (or ricotta), parsley, and garlic.

Pour 1 cup of sauce in bottom of pan. Layer in this order:

4 noodles, 1/2 cheese mixture, 1/2 mozzarella, 1 cup sauce, 4 noodles, 1/2 cheese mixture, 1/2 mozzarella, 1 cup sauce, 4 noodles, and the rest of the sauce. Sprinkle with Parmesan cheese. Covered tightly with aluminum foil and bake for 1 hour. Increase baking time by 15 minutes if it has been refrigerated.

Or one jar (1 pound, 10 ounces) and water to equal 4 cups.

Nutrition note: Great source of dairy and protein, not to mention it is quick and easy!

Per serving: 218 calories, 5 g fat, 2 g saturated fat, 28 g carbohydrate, 15 g protein, 9 mg cholesterol, 596 mg sodium, 2 g dietary fiber, 6 g sugar

Source: © 2008 Brenda J. Ponichtera–*www.quickandhealthy.net*
From *Quick & Healthy Recipes and Ideas, 3rd Edition*
Reprinted with permission from Small Steps Press

Balsamic-Glazed Salmon
Makes 4 servings

4 4-oz. salmon filets
1 cup balsamic vinegar
2 tsp. canola or olive oil

Marinate salmon filets in the balsamic vinegar for 1 hour.

Heat the oil in a sauté pan over medium/medium-high heat.

Remove the salmon from the marinade (reserving remaining) and cook in sauté pan, skin side up, for 3 to 4 minutes. Flip (adding oil if needed) and cook 3 to 4 minutes more or until cooked through.

Remove salmon, add balsamic marinade to pan, cook 2 to 5 minutes or until beginning to thicken and reduced by half. Pour balsamic glaze over salmon, serve, and enjoy!

Serving suggestions:

Serve over whole-wheat pasta with pesto and your favorite veggies (broccoli, tomatoes, asparagus, spinach, etc.).

Or pair with a side of your favorite veggies and a whole grain such as brown rice.

Nutrition note: Salmon is loaded with healthy omega-3 fats and is low in mercury content.

Per serving: 270 calories, 14 g fat, 3 g saturated fat, 6 g monounsaturated fat, 5 g polyunsaturated fat, 8 g carbohydrate, 23 g protein, 65 mg cholesterol, 85 mg sodium, 0 g dietary fiber

Source: Allison Stevens MS, RD, LD
Healthy Living, Healthy Flavors LLC
www.healthylivinghealthyflavors.com

Slow Cooker
Middle Eastern Stew

Makes 6 servings

1/4 cup olive oil
8 boneless, skinless chicken thighs, cut into 1-inch cubes
1 eggplant, peeled, cut into 2-inch cubes
3 onions, peeled and thinly sliced
4 carrots, peeled and thinly sliced
4 cloves garlic, peeled and minced
1/2 cup dried cranberries
2 cups reduced-sodium chicken broth
2 Tbs. tomato paste
2 Tbs. lemon juice
2 Tbs. all-purpose flour
1 1/2 tsp. ground cumin
1 1/2 tsp. ground ginger
1 1/2 tsp. ground cinnamon
1 cup water

In a heavy skillet, heat half the olive oil over medium-high heat. Add half the chicken to pan and brown on all sides. Do not cook all the way through. Repeat with the remaining oil and chicken. Place browned chicken in the bottom of a slow cooker. Place eggplant, onions, carrots, garlic, and cranberries over the chicken.

In a medium bowl, place the chicken broth, tomato paste, lemon juice, flour, cumin, ginger, cinnamon, and water. Whisk together until blended thoroughly. Pour the mixture into the slow cooker. Cook on high for 5 hours. Serve with whole-wheat couscous and a green salad.

Nutrition note: Great source of fiber, veggies, and protein, with a dose of folate and choline, both important to stock up on before and during pregnancy.

Per serving: 331 calories, 21 g fat, 21 g carbohydrates, 16 g protein, 64 mg cholesterol, 275 mg sodium, 5 g dietary fiber, 50 mg calcium, 43 mcg folate, 2 mg iron, 56 mg choline.

Source: Elizabeth M. Ward, MS, RD
www.expectthebestpregnancy.com

Stir-Fried Vegetables with Edamame

Makes 6 servings

2 Tbs. olive oil
1 tsp. cumin seeds
3 cloves garlic, chopped
1/2 jalapeno pepper, sliced in half
1 1/2 cups corn kernels, fresh
1/4 tsp. turmeric
1/4 tsp. salt or to taste
1 cup frozen edamame, thawed (young green soybeans)
3 cups cut zucchini, fresh
1 cup cut sweet red bell pepper, fresh
1 cup chopped (with tender stems) cilantro
Juice of 1/2 a lemon

Add jalapeno, salt, and turmeric to the corn.

Heat a 3-quart skillet or pan on medium-high heat with 1 teaspoon cumin seeds. When the seeds begin to change color and give off an aroma, add 2 tablespoons olive oil and the chopped garlic, and turn heat to medium.

Fry the garlic for a minute and add the corn with jalapeno salt and turmeric. Stir and cook covered for 2 to 3 minutes. Stir in edamame, zucchini, and red pepper. Stir and cook covered for 3 to 4 minutes. Before serving, add chopped cilantro and fresh lemon juice, and stir to mix all the ingredients.

Serve the vegetables over rice, quinoa, chicken, or fish, or for lunch in a pita pocket.

Nutrition note: A great source of plant protein with a good dose of fiber, calcium, and healthy fats.

Per serving: 163 calories, 8 g fat, 1 g saturated fat, 4 g monounsaturated fat, 2 g polyunsaturated fat, 18 g carbohydrate, 8 g protein, 0 mg cholesterol, 119 mg sodium, 4 g dietary fiber, 112 mg calcium, 2.5 mg iron, 116 mcg folate

Source: Gita Patel, MS, RD, CDE, LD, CLT
www.feedinghealth.com

Eggs Florentine Wrap
Makes 1 serving

2 eggs

1 oz. feta cheese

1 cup fresh baby spinach, packed, roughly chopped

1/4 medium onion, diced

1 Tbs. tub margarine

1 medium (7 or 8 inches) whole-wheat tortilla

Salt and fresh ground black pepper, to taste

In a medium bowl, beat eggs. Add cheese and set aside. Heat a large skillet over medium heat. Add half the margarine. Add onions and cook until transparent. Add spinach to the pan and cook until just wilted, about one minute. Place onion and spinach mixture in a small bowl and set aside. Add remaining butter to skillet, lower heat to medium-low, and add the egg and cottage cheese mixture. Using a heat-proof spatula, gently scramble egg mixture until cooked. Add spinach and onion mixture back to pan and mix with eggs. Place this mixture in the center of the tortilla, fold in the sides, then roll up.

Nutrition note: Great source of fiber, folate, and iron, not to mention protein and choline (all important to fertility and pregnancy).

Per serving: 384 calories, 21 **g** fat, 27 g carbohydrate, 21 g protein, 448 mg cholesterol, 805 mg sodium, 4 g dietary fiber, 281 mg calcium, 162 mcg folate, 5 mg iron, 625 mg choline

Source: Elizabeth M. Ward, MS, RD

www.expectthebestpregnancy.com

Salmon in a Crunch
Makes 8 servings

2 pounds salmon filet

1 1/2 Tbs. mustard

1 tsp. horseradish sauce
1 tsp. reduced-fat mayonnaise
1 Tbs. balsamic vinegar
1 Tbs. lemon juice or the juice of a 1/2 fresh lemon
1 Tbs. fresh chopped parsley or dill, to taste
Freshly ground pepper, to taste
1 Tbs. sliced almonds
Lemon slices (for garnish)
Cooking spray (Pam)

Preheat oven to 375.

Line a cookie sheet with foil wrap and spray with cooking spray.

Place salmon, skin side down, on prepared cookie sheet.

In a small bowl, combine mustard, horseradish sauce, mayonnaise, balsamic vinegar, lemon juice, parsley or dill, and pepper. Spread evenly over salmon.

Lightly sprinkle sliced almonds evenly over salmon.

Bake salmon on the middle rack in the oven for 45 minutes or until salmon is opaque in center.

Transfer to platter and garnish with lemon wedges.

Nutrition note: This tasty recipe will provide you with a load of protein as well as healthy fats, including omega-3 fats.

Per serving: 225 calories, 11 g fat, 1.8 g saturated fat, 3.6 g monounsaturated fat, 4 g polyunsaturated fat, 1.2 g carbohydrates, 29 g protein, 82 mg cholesterol, 112 mg sodium, 0.2 g dietary fiber, 0.5 g sugar, 24 g calcium, 35 g folate, 1.3 g iron

Source: Bonnie Taub-Dix, MA, RD, CDN

Owner, BTD Nutrition Consultants, LLC, *www.bonnietaubdix.co*

Side Dishes/Salads

 Sweet Potato Quinoa

Makes 5, 1 1/3-cup servings for a meal or 10, 2/3-cup servings as a side dish.

1 cup dry quinoa
2 cups water
2 cups roasted sweet potato fries, diced (recipe follows)
1 15-oz. can organic black beans, no added salt (rinsed and drained)
1 cup frozen corn kernels, thawed
1 cup diced red bell pepper
3 scallions, finely chopped
2 Tbs. chopped fresh parsley
3 Tbs. extra-virgin olive oil, divided
Freshly squeezed lemon juice to taste
1/2 cup crumbled low-fat feta cheese
Salt and pepper to taste

Note: Make roasted sweet potatoes the night before and store in the refrigerator for super easy preparation.

Rinse and drain quinoa well.

In a saucepan, combine quinoa, water, and a pinch of salt. Bring to a boil, reduce heat, cover, and simmer for 15 to 20 minutes, until water is absorbed and quinoa is tender. Once quinoa is cooked, transfer to a large bowl, stir in 1 Tbs. of olive oil, and set aside to cool.

In a separate bowl combine sweet potatoes, black beans, corn, bell pepper, scallions, and parsley. Toss to combine.

Combine sweet potato mixture with quinoa; add remaining oil, lemon juice, and feta. Season with salt and pepper to taste. Toss and serve chilled or at room temperature.

Sweet Potato Fries

1 Tbs. olive oil
2 medium sweet potatoes
Salt and pepper

Preheat oven to 425.

Cut 2 medium sweet potatoes into 1/2-inch thick fries.

Lay potatoes on a sheet pan. Toss with 1 Tbs. olive oil, salt, and pepper.Bake for 30 to 40 minutes or until golden brown, turning once half way through roasting.

Nutrition note: Great plant protein source, full of healthy fats, calcium, fiber, folate, and iron, all needed to help boost fertility.

Per serving: 346 calories, 10 g fat, 1 g saturated fat, 35 g carbohydrates, 11 g protein, 0 mg cholesterol, 96 mg sodium, 10.5 g dietary fiber, 78 mg calcium, 96 mcg folate, 4 mg iron

Source: Dana Angelo White, MS, RD, ATC

Owner, Dana White Nutrition, Inc.

www.danawhitenutrition.com

 ## Sweet Tropics Fruit Salad
Make 8 servings

1 large stalk of celery, cut into 1/2-inch cubes
3 golden kiwi fruits, peeled and cut into 1/2-inch cubes
2 chayote squash, peeled and cut into 1/2-inch cubes
1 medium orange, peeled and cut into segments
1/4 cup finely minced red onion
1 medium mango (ripe but still firm), peeled and cut into
    1/2-inch cubes
1 jalapeno pepper, seeded and finely minced
3 Tbs. fresh lemon juice
1 tsp. extra-virgin olive oil
4 Tbs. finely chopped fresh mint leaves

Peel and chop ingredients as directed. Combine ingredients in a large bowl and mix well. Add salt to taste.

Nutrition note: Perfect dish to get in your fruits and vegetables and all the fertility boosting nutrients they contain. Provides a good dose of fiber, as well!

Per serving: 70 calories, 2 g fat, 0 g saturated fat, 14 g carbohydrates, 1 g protein, 0 mg cholesterol, 10 mg sodium, 3 g dietary fiber, 9 g sugar

Source: Chef Stephanie Green, RD

Nutrition Studio

www.nutritionstudio.com

Lucy's Taboule Salad

Makes 10 servings

1 package Near East brand Taboule Wheat Salad Mix
1/2 pint grape tomatoes, sliced in half
1/2 medium cucumber, peeled and chopped
1/2 cup black olives, sliced
3 Tbs. olive oil
1 1/2 Tbs. lemon juice
2 Tbs. fresh mint, finely chopped
1/2 cup crumbled feta cheese

This recipe was adapted from the recipe of John's mother, Lucy. She was of Lebanese decent and prepared this dish often. It's great as a summertime side dish, or "snick snack," as Lucy would say!

Combine Near East wheat mix and spice package in large bowl. Add 1 cup boiling water and stir. Cover and refrigerate for 30 minutes.

Stir in tomatoes, cucumber, olives, olive oil, lemon juice, mint, and feta cheese.

Refrigerate 1 to 2 hours prior to serving.

Nutrition note: A tasty way to include whole grains and veggies, not to mention fiber and healthy fats.

Per serving (2/3 cup): 115 calories, 7 g fat, 1.5 g saturated fat, 3.5 g monounsaturated , 0.6 g polyunsaturated fat, 13 g carbohydrates, 3 g protein, 4 mg cholesterol, 250 mg sodium, 3 g dietary fiber, 35 mg calcium

Source: Angie and John Lamberson
Nutrition Pair, LLC
www.nutritionpair.com

Bulgur Delight

Makes 4 servings

1/2 cup bulgur wheat
1 cup strong green tea
3 medium tomatoes, seeded and diced

1 Tbs. olive oil
4 clove garlic, finely minced
1 tsp. salt
Freshly ground pepper
1 1/2 cups minced greens such as parsley, arugula, or mint
6 scallions, chopped
1 medium cucumber, peeled, seeded, and diced
1/4 cup fresh lemon juice
1 cup water

Place bulgur in a bowl.

Heat water and steep tea 3 to 4 minutes. Add to bulgur and allow to soak for 10 minutes. Drain off remaining liquid.

Place tomatoes, olive oil, garlic, salt, and pepper in a bowl and allow to marinate for about 30 minutes. Combine all remaining ingredients and mix well.

Nutrition note: Great source of whole grains and fiber. Includes green tea, which is chock full of antioxidants and is said to help boost fertility.

Per serving: 130 calories, 4 g fat, 0.5 g saturated fat, 23 g carbohydrate, 4 g protein, 0 mg cholesterol, 600 mg sodium, 5 g dietary fiber, 4 g sugar

Source: Chef Stephanie Green, RD

Nutrition Studio

www.nutritionstudio.com

 # Honey Glazed Baby Carrots and Radishes

Makes 4 to 6 servings

1 Tbs. olive oil
1 small shallot, finely diced
1/2 tsp. dried thyme leaves
1/4 tsp. ground marjoram
1/2 lb. baby carrots
1/2 lb. radishes, halved

2 Tbs. honey
3/4 tsp. kosher salt

In a large pan over medium heat, combine olive oil, shallot, thyme, and marjoram. Cook for about one minute. Add carrots and radishes and cook for about five minutes, constantly stirring. Add honey and salt and stir to coat.

Nutrition Note: If you count on baby carrots to help boost your conception chances, this is another delicious way to add them to your diet. It also adds the possible fertility boosting properties of honey.

Per serving: 120 calories, 3.5 g fat, 0.5 g saturated fat, 20 g carbohydrates, 2 g protein, 0 mg cholesterol, 410 mg sodium, 2 g dietary fiber, 13 g sugar

Source: Chef Stephanie Green, RD
Nutrition Studio
www.nutritionstudio.com

 ## Crispy Baked Asparagus
Makes 4 servings

2 bunches asparagus, washed (about one lb. per bunch)
1 Tbs. extra virgin olive oil
Salt and cracked black pepper to taste

Preheat oven to 400 degrees F. Snap off the thick bottom portion of the asparagus stalks (about 1–2 inches) and discard. Place the asparagus in a large plastic bag. Drizzle the olive oil, salt, and cracked black pepper over the asparagus, seal the bag, and shake to evenly coat the asparagus with the olive oil and to distribute the salt and cracked black pepper. Refrigerate until ready to bake. Place the asparagus in a single layer on a non-stick cookie sheet (*discarding* any extra oil that is left in the bag). Bake approximately 15 to 20 minutes or until slightly crispy. Serve.

Nutrition note: What a tasty way to add fiber and healthy fats, not to mention vegetables, to your diet.

Per serving: 65 calories, 4 g fat, 0.5 g saturated fat, 2.75 g mono-unsaturated fat, 0.25 g polyunsaturated fat, 5 g carbohydrates, 5 g protein, 152 mg sodium, 4.7 g dietary fiber, 42 mg calcium: 42 milligrams.

Source: Joey Mock, RD, LD

Healthy Habitudes, LLC

www.healthyhabitudes.com

Soups/Chili

 ## Chicken Chili

Makes 5, 1 1/4-cup servings

1/2 lb. skinless, boneless chicken breasts
3/4 cup chopped onion
2 tsp. chopped garlic
2 cans (15 ounces each) kidney beans, drained and rinsed
1 can (14.5 ounces) diced tomatoes, not drained
1 can (4 ounces) diced green chilies
1 cup water
1 Tbs. dried cilantro
2 tsp. chili powder
1/2 tsp. ground cumin

Cut chicken in bite-size pieces. Brown chicken in a saucepan that has been sprayed with non-stick cooking spray. Add remaining ingredients. Cover and simmer for 30 minutes or until chicken is tender.

Nutrition note: One serving is an excellent source of fiber and protein yet low in fat.

Per serving: 236 calories, 2 g fat, 0 g saturated fat, 33 g carbohydrates, 21 g protein, 28 mg cholesterol, 64 mg sodium, 10 g dietary fiber, 3 g sugar

Source: © 2009 Brenda J. Ponichtera—*www.quickandhealthy.net*

From *Quick & Healthy Volume II, 2nd Edition*

Reprinted with permission from Small Steps Press

Curry Shrimp Chowder

Makes 6 servings

1 Tbs. extra-virgin olive oil
1 medium red onion, chopped
1 medium bell pepper, chopped
1/2 cup celery, chopped
3 garlic cloves, minced
2 Tbs. ginger, minced
1/4 tsp. kosher salt
1 Tbs. curry powder
1 cup canned tomato sauce
3 1/2 cups low-sodium or homemade chicken or vegetable broth
3 Tbs. crunchy or creamy almond butter
1 lb. raw shrimp, peeled, deveined, and cut into bite-sized chunks
1 1/2 cups frozen edamame
3 cups baby spinach or other chopped fresh greens

Heat olive oil in a large soup pot or Dutch oven. Add onion, bell pepper, and celery, sauté until softened, about 5 minutes. Add garlic, ginger, salt, curry powder; cook for an additional 3 minutes. Add tomato sauce and broth and bring to a simmer. Whisk in almond butter until well blended. Add seafood and edamame, cook until heated through. Allow stew to simmer for about 15 minutes (or longer if desired). Stir in parley and spinach.

Nutrition note: Excellent source of healthy omega-3 fats, not to mention calcium and fiber. This dish packs a protein punch, as well.

Per serving: 327 calories, 16 g fat, 2 g saturated fat, 620 mg omega-3 fats, 20 g carbohydrates, 27 g protein, 120 mg cholesterol, 634 mg sodium, 4 g dietary fiber, 161 mg calcium, 30 mcg folate, 5 mg iron

Source: Dana Angelo White, MS, RD, ATC
Owner, Dana White Nutrition, Inc.
www.danawhitenutrition.com

Butternut Squash Soup
Makes 4 servings

2 Tbs. olive oil
1 medium onion, chopped
2 cups squash
1 medium potato, diced
2 1/2 cups non-fat chicken broth
Salt and pepper, to taste

Preheat oven to 350. Cut butternut squash in half and scoop out seeds. Place cut side down on a foil lined pan. Bake for 45 to 60 minutes or until fork tender. Let cool and scoop out the squash. Leftovers may be frozen and used at another time. Heat olive oil in a large saucepan, add onions, and cook for 5 minutes until softened. Add potato and cook for 5 minutes. Add the squash and chicken broth and bring to a boil. Turn down the heat; cover and simmer for about 30 minutes. Puree mixture in a blender. Return mixture to saucepan and reheat. Taste and season well with salt, pepper, and lemon juice.

Nutrition note: Great source of fiber and healthy fats, not to mention plenty of antioxidants!

Per serving: 160 calories, 7 g fat, 1 g saturated fat, 22 g carbohydrates, 3 g protein, 0 mg cholesterol, 590 mg sodium, 4 g dietary fiber, 4 g sugar

Source: Chef Stephanie Green, RD
Nutrition Studio
www.nutritionstudio.com

Lentil Soup
Makes 8 servings

1 lb. lentils (can use red lentils)
12 cups water
4 Tbs. olive oil

1 onion, chopped
4 carrots, chopped
1 tomato, chopped, or 1 can tomatoes, drained
3 or 4 cloves garlic, crushed
3 or 4 bay leaves
Salt and pepper to taste
Optional: chopped spinach leaves*

Wash lentils and drain. Heat oil in pot. Add onion and sauté. Add all other ingredients (except water), lentils last. Add water and bring to boil. Reduce heat, cover, and simmer 30 to 45 minutes until lentils are soft (not mushy). Remove bay leaves.

*Add spinach just before serving.

Nutrition note: This delicious soup is loaded with fertility boosting nutrients including fiber, plant protein, folate, and healthy fats.

Per serving: 150 calories, 7 g fat, 5 g monounsaturated fat, 0.8 g polyunsaturated fat, 0.9 g saturated fat, 17 g carbohydrates, 6 g protein, 0 mg cholesterol, 160 mg sodium, 6.5 g dietary fiber, 3 g sugar, 41 mg calcium, 2.7 mg iron, 114 mg folate

Source: Faye Berger Mitchell, RD, LD

Nutritionist in Private Practice in Bethesda, Maryland

www.fayethenutritionist.com

Dips/Spreads

 Peanut Butter Yogurt Dip
Makes 10 servings

2 cups (16oz) nonfat Greek yogurt
1/4 cup peanut butter
1/2 tsp. vanilla extract
1/4 tsp. cinnamon
2 Tbs. pure maple syrup

Place all ingredients in a medium bowl and use a fork to combine until mixed well.

Serving suggestions:

- Use as a dip for your favorite sliced fruit: bananas, strawberries, apples, and more!
- Use instead of butter and syrup (refined sugar) to top whole grain waffles or pancakes.

Storage:

- Keep the yogurt container and use to store the dip.
- Keep refrigerated for up to 1 week.

Nutrition note: Peanut butter contains healthy fats. Friendly bacteria or probiotics from yogurt is essential to good health.

Per serving: 60 calories, 3 g fat, 0.5 saturated fat, 1.5 g mono-unsaturated fat, 1 g polyunsaturated fat, 5 g carbohydrates, 4 g protein, 0 mg cholesterol, 10 mg sodium, 1 g dietary fiber, 40 mg calcium

Source: Allison Stevens MS, RD, LD
Healthy Living, Healthy Flavors LLC
www.healthylivinghealthyflavors.com

 ## Sweet and Spicy Hummus
Serves: 15

2 (15 oz.) cans chickpeas
3 Tbs. sesame tahini
1 Tbs. honey
1/4 cup extra-virgin olive oil
Juice of 1/2 a lemon
1/4 cup fresh basil leaves
1/4 tsp. chili powder
1/4 tsp. ground cumin
1/4 tsp. paprika
1/4 tsp. kosher salt
Freshly ground black pepper, to taste

Rinse and drain chickpeas. Combine ingredients in a food processor and pulse until smooth. Serve with fresh vegetables and/or pita chips.

Nutrition note: A great source of plant protein and healthy omega-3 fats.

Per serving: 102 calories, 5.5 g fat, 0.5 g saturated fat, 10 mg omega-3 fats, 10 g carbohydrates, 3.5 g protein, 0 mg cholesterol, 34 mg sodium, 2 g dietary fiber, 38 mg calcium, 4 mcg folate, 0.7 mg iron

Source: Dana Angelo White, MS, RD, ATC

Owner, Dana White Nutrition, Inc.

www.danawhitenutrition.com

 ## Lemon Cannellini Spread
Makes 4 servings

2 large garlic cloves

1 can (15 oz.) white kidney beans, drained

1 Tbs. olive oil

1 Tbs. lemon juice

1 tsp. lemon zest

1/4 tsp. kosher salt

Pepper, to taste

Into a food processor add the garlic cloves and pulse until the garlic is chopped. Add the remaining ingredients. Let the food processor run for about a minute to develop a very creamy spread. Serve with crackers or your favorite vegetable.

Nutrition note: The perfect dip to give your veggies a zip. A great source of fiber, calcium, and plant protein.

Per serving: 133 calories, 4g fat, 18 g carbohydrates, 7 g protein, 8g dietary fiber, 9 g sugar, 85 mg calcium

Source: Chef Stephanie Green, RD

Nutrition Studio, *www.nutritionstudio.com*

Smoothies/Shakes

Pineapple Smoothie
Makes one serving

1/2 medium banana, sliced and frozen (freeze ahead of time)

1/2 cup frozen pineapple chunks

1/4 cup nonfat Greek-style yogurt

1/2 cup orange juice

1/4 cup water

Combine ingredients in a blender. Blend until smooth.

Nutrition note: Great source of calcium, folate, and omega-3 fats, needed for good overall and fertility health. Also includes possible cervical mucus–producing pineapple.

Per serving: 176 calories, 0.5 g fat, 0 g saturated fat, 20 mg omega-3 fats, 38 g carbohydrates, 7 g protein, 0 mg cholesterol, 25 mg sodium, 3 g dietary fiber, 95 mg calcium, 61 mcg folate, 0.6 mg iron

Source: Dana Angelo White, MS, RD, ATC

Owner, Dana White Nutrition, Inc.

www.danawhitenutrition.com

"Banilla" Shake
Makes one serving

1/2 medium banana, sliced and frozen (freeze ahead of time)

3/4 cup low-fat milk

1 Tbs. honey

1 tsp. pure vanilla extract

4 to 5 ice cubes

Combine ingredients in a blender. Blend until smooth.

Nutrition note: Excellent source of calcium and sweetened with fertility-boosting honey.

Per serving: 211 calories, 2 g fat, 1 g saturated fat, 41 g carbohydrates, 7 g protein, 11 mg cholesterol, 95 mg sodium, 1.5 g dietary fiber, 230 mg calcium, 12 mcg folate, 0.25 mg iron

Source: Dana Angelo White, MS, RD, ATC

Owner, Dana White Nutrition, Inc.

www.danawhitenutrition.com

 Pumpkin Smoothie
Makes one serving

1/2 cup milk

1/2 cup canned pumpkin puree

1 tsp. vanilla extract

1 tsp. brown sugar

Pinch of cinnamon

2 ice cubes

In a food processor or blender, combine milk, canned pumpkin puree, vanilla extract, brown sugar, pinch of cinnamon, and ice cubes. Process until frothy and enjoy immediately.

Nutrition Note: Perfect way to get in your calcium and add a bunch of antioxidants for top fertility health.

Per serving: 110 calories, 2 g fat, 21 g carbohydrates, 5 g protein, 6 mg cholesterol, 61 mg sodium, 4 g dietary fiber, 181 mg calcium, 21 mcg folate, 34 mg choline

Source: Elizabeth M. Ward, MS, RD

www.expectthebestpregnancy.com

Breads/Muffins

 ## Banana-Almond Bread/Muffins
Makes 2 loaves or 24 muffins

1 cup whole-wheat pastry flour
2 1/3 cups all-purpose flour
1 Tbs. baking powder
2 tsp. baking soda
1 tsp. salt
1 tsp. ground cinnamon
1 1/2 cups granulated sugar
4 egg whites
1/2 cup canola oil
1/2 cup skim milk
1/2 tsp. lemon juice
1 tsp. pure vanilla extract
2 large eggs
2/3 cup water
4 ripe bananas, mashed well
1/3 cup chopped almonds
Cooking spray

Preheat oven to 350.

Spoon flours into dry measuring cups and level with a knife. Whisk together with baking powder, baking soda, salt, and cinnamon in a large bowl.

Combine milk and lemon juice and let stand.

Combine sugar, egg whites, oil, vanilla extract, and eggs in a large bowl and beat with a hand mixer at a high speed until blended.

Add milk/lemon juice to sugar mixture.

Add water and mashed bananas, beating at a low speed until blended together.

Add flower mixture and beat at a low speed just until combined (don't overmix.)

Coat 2 loaf pans (9 x 5-inch each) or muffin tins (24 muffins) with cooking spray.

Spoon batter into pans and fill halfway. Sprinkle almonds evenly over batter.

Bake bread (in loaf pans) for 1 hour or until a wooden pick inserted in center comes out clean, or bake muffins (in muffin tins) for 30 minutes and check as above.

Cool in pans for 10 minutes and then remove from pans and cool on wire rack.

Nutrition Note: Full of healthy fats, some protein, calcium, and folate, and the possible fertility-boosting powers of bananas.

Per serving (per muffin): 187 calories, 6 g fat, 0.6 saturated fat, 3.5 g monounsaturated fat, 1.7 g polyunsaturated fat, 30 g carbohydrates, 4 g protein, 15 mg cholesterol, 269 mg sodium, 1.7 g dietary fiber, 15 g sugar, 47 mg calcium, 31 mcg folate

Source: Bonnie Taub-Dix, MA, RD, CDN

Owner, BTD Nutrition Consultants, LLC

www.bonnietaubdix.com

Simple Seven-Day Meal Plan

*Recipe included

Day One

Breakfast:

Whole-wheat toast w/ omega-3 peanut butter
Sliced strawberries
Hot caffeine-free green tea w/ honey

Mid-Morning:

Low-fat fruit yogurt
Fresh blueberries

Lunch:

*Sweet and Spicy Hummus
Baby carrots, celery sticks, and red pepper slices
Whole-wheat crackers

Mid-Day:

*Pineapple smoothie

Dinner:

*Chicken Chili
Green salad and raw veggies topped with vinegar and
olive oil dressing
Glass of milk

Evening Snack:

Air-popped popcorn

Day Two

Breakfast:

Oatmeal topped with blueberries and almonds
Glass of milk
Hot caffeine-free green tea w/ honey

Mid-Morning:

Low-fat cheese
Whole-wheat crackers

Lunch:

*Lentil Soup
Green salad w/ vinegar and olive oil dressing

Mid-Day:

Apple topped with Omega-3 peanut butter

Dinner:

*Salmon in a Crunch
Brown rice

*Crispy Baked Asparagus
Glass of milk

Evening Snack:

*Peanut Butter Yogurt Dip
Fresh fruit

Day Three

Breakfast:

*Eggs Florentine Wrap
Cantaloupe cubes
Glass of milk

Mid-Morning:

Low-fat yogurt
Walnuts

Lunch:

Tuna salad and sliced avocado on whole-wheat pita bread
Red pepper slices
Kiwi fruit

Mid-Day:

Baby carrots and celery sticks
*Lemon Cannellini Spread

Dinner:

*Slow Cooker Middle Eastern Stew
Whole-wheat couscous
Green salad and raw veggies w/ vinegar and olive oil
    dressing

Evening Snack:

Handful of peanuts

Day Four

Breakfast:
> Whole-grain cereal w/ milk
> Red grapefruit
> Hot caffeine-free green tea w/ honey

Mid-Morning:
> Almonds
> Raisins

Lunch:
> *Lucy's Taboule Salad
> Kiwi fruit

Mid-Day:
> Fresh orange
> *Banana-Almond Muffin

Dinner:
> *Quick Lasagna
> Green salad and raw veggies topped with vinegar and
>   olive oil dressing
> Glass of milk

Evening Snack:
> Air-popped popcorn

Day Five

Breakfast:
> *"Banilla" Shake
> Whole-wheat English muffin topped with almond butter

Mid-Morning:
> Red pepper strips
> *Sweet and Spicy Hummus

Lunch:

Grilled chicken, tomato salsa, sliced avocado in whole-wheat pita

Grapes

Mid-Day:

*Pumpkin Smoothie

Dinner:

*Curry Shrimp Chowder

Whole-wheat couscous

Glass of milk

Evening Snack:

Cinnamon baked apple

Chopped walnuts

Day Six

Breakfast:

Omelet w/ cheddar cheese, green pepper, tomato, and onion

Whole-wheat toast topped with almond butter

Glass of milk

Mid-Morning:

Kiwi fruit

Hot caffeine-free green tea w/ honey

Lunch:

*Lentil Soup

Green salad w/ vinegar and olive oil dressing

Whole-wheat crackers

Mid-Day:

Baby carrots and celery

*Lemon Cannellini Spread

Dinner:

Grilled chicken breast
*Sweet Potato Quinoa
Glass of milk

Evening Snack:

*Peanut Butter Yogurt Dip
Fresh fruit

Day Seven

Breakfast:

Oatmeal topped w/ strawberries, raisins and cinnamon
Glass of milk

Mid-Morning:

Apple topped w/ Omega-3 peanut butter

Lunch:

*Butternut Squash Soup
*Banana-Almond Muffin
Fresh orange

Mid-Day:

*Pineapple Smoothie

Dinner:

*Stir Fried Vegetables With Edamame
Brown rice
Green salad and raw veggies topped with vinegar and
    olive oil dressing
Glass of milk

Evening Snack:

Handful of peanuts

Raisins

Resources

Body Mass Index

National Heart, Lung, and Blood Institute/National Institutes of Health: *www.nhlbisupport.com/bmi*

Center for Disease Control and Prevention: *www.cdc. gov/healthyweight/assessing/bmi*

Books

Elizabeth Ward, MS, RD

Expect the Best: Your Guide to Healthy Eating Before, During, and After Pregnancy (Wiley, 2009)
www.expectthebestpregnancy.com

April Rudat, MS Ed, RD, LDN

Oh Yes You Can Breastfeed Twins! Plus More Tips for Simplifying Life with Twins (April Rudat, Registered Dietitian LLC, 2007)
www.ohyesyoucanbreastfeedtwins.com

Bridget Swinney, MS, RD

Eating Expectantly (Meadowbrook Press, 2000), *Baby Bites* (Meadowbrook Press, 2007), *Healthy Food for Healthy Kids* (Meadowbrook Press, 1999), *www.healthyfoodzone.com*

Brenda J. Poinchtera, RD

Quick & Healthy Recipes and Ideas (Small Steps Press, 2008). To order this book, please call 1-800-232-6733 or order online at *www.shopdiabetes.org.*

Quick & Healthy Volume II, 2nd Edition (Small Steps Press, 2009). To order this book, please call 1-800-232-6455 or order online at *www.shopdiabetes.org.*

Celiac Disease

Tell Me What to Eat If I Have Celiac Disease (Career Press, 2009), Kimberly A. Tessmer, RD, LD

National Digestive Diseases Information Clearinghouse (NDDIC): *http://digestive.niddk.nih.gov/ddiseases/pubs/celiac/*

Celiac Disease Foundation: *www.celiac.org*

Celiac.com: *www.celiac.com*

Celiac Sprue Assocation: *www.csaceliacs.org*

National Foundation for Celiac Awareness: *www.celiaccentral.org*

Complementary and Alternative Medicine

Acupuncture

National Certification Commission for Acupuncture and Oriental Medicine: *www.nccaom.org*

American Academy of Medical Acupuncture: *www.medicalacupuncture.org*

Acupuncture.com: *www.acupunture.com*

Herbs/Dietary Supplements

National Center for Complimentary and Alternative Medicine: *http://nccam.nih.gov/health/supplements/wiseuse.htm*

Natural Medicines Comprehensive Database: *http://naturaldatabase.therapeuticresearch.com/nd/Search.aspx?s=ND&cs=&pt=1&rli=1&anchor=basic#basic*

National Institutes for Health, Office of Dietary Supplements: http://ods.od.nih.gov/

United States National Library of Medicine, Dietary Supplements Labels Database: *http://dietarysupplements.nlm.nih.gov/dietary/*

Herb Research Foundation: *www.herbs.org*

Herbs at a Glance: A Quick Guide to Herbal Supplements (National Center for Complementary and Alternative Medicine): *http://nccam.nih.gov/health/NIH_Herbs_at_a_Glance.pdf*

Reiki

International Association of Reiki Professionals: *www.iarp.org*

The International Center for Reiki Training: *www.reiki.org.*

Yoga

Yoga Journal: *www.yogajournal.com*

Yoga Basics: *www.yogabasics.com*

Eating Disorders

National Eating Disorders Association: *www. nationaleatingdisorders.org/*

Eating Disorder Referral and Information Center: *wwwedreferral.com*

National Association of Anorexia Nervosa and Associated Disorders: *www.anad.org*

Endometriosis

The Endometriosis Association: *www.endo-online.org*

The Hormone Foundation: *www.hormone.org*

Endometriosis.org: *www.endometriosis.org*

Fertility-Based Websites

Resolve- The National Infertility Association: *www.resolve.org*

American Society for Reproductive Medicine: *www.asrm.org*

Womenshealth.gov: *http://womenshealth.gov/pregnancy/ before-you-get-pregnant/preconception-health.cfm*

Center for Applied Reproductive Science (CARS): *www.ivf-et.com*

InterNational Council on Infertility Information
Dissemination, Inc. (INCIID): *www.inciid.org*
Fertility Friend: *www.fertilityfriend.com*
Baby Center: *www.babycenter.com*
The American Congress of Obstetricians and
 Gynccologists: *http://www.acog.org*
March of Dimes: *www.marchofdimes.com*
Society for Fetal-Maternal Medicine: *www.smfm.org*

Food and Nutrition

American Dietetic Association: *www.eatright.org*

American Heart Association: *www. americanheart.org*

United States Department of Agriculture/
ChooseMyPlate.gov: *www.choosemyplate.gov*

Dietary Guidelines for Americans: *www.health.gov/*
 dietaryguidelines

U.S. FDA Labeling and Nutrition: *www.fda.gov/Food/*
LabelingNutrition

National Organic Program: *http://www.ams.usda.*
 govAMSv1.0/nop

Environmental Working Group: *http://www.foodnews.org*

United States Environmental Protection Agency/Fish
 Advisories: *www.epa.gov/ost/fish*

American Heart Association: *www.americanheart.org*

The Vegetarian Resource Group: *www.vrg.org*

Vegetarian Times: *www.vegetariantimes.com*

PCOS

Women's Health Research, National Institute of Child
 Health and Human Development (NICHD), NIH,
 HHS: *www.nichd.nih.gov/womenshealth*

Polycystic Ovarian Syndrome Association, Inc.
(PCOSA): *www.pcosupport.org*
PCOS NutritioCenter:*www.pcos nutrition.com*

Practitioners Specializing In Fertility/Women's Health

Sadhana Bienzen, MS, RD, CD

Smart Results, LLC. Specializing in autism, ADHD, cardiovascular disease, celiac disease, child and family nutrition, food allergies, gastro-intestinal disorders, vegetarian nutrition, weight management, and women's health (PCOS, in-fertility, pregnancy, lactation, menopause).

sbienzen@hotmail.com

414-467-7947

Fax: 414-423-8140

Franklin, WI 53132

Amber Wilson, MS, RD

NewBaby Nutrition. Specializing in individual and couples counseling, writing, and speaking on the topic of TTC, pregnant women, and families.

www.newbabynutrition.com

Bay Area and Sacramento, CA

Gita Patel, MS, RD, CDE, LD, CLT

Vegetarian diabetes educator, certified LEAP therapist, author, consultant, speaker. Specializing in IBS, migraine, and other inflammatory conditions often triggered by delayed food hypersensitivities.

www.feedinghealth.com

gita@feedinghealth.com

Cheryl Harris, MPH, RD, CLC

Harris Whole Health

Alexandria, VA

www.harriswholehealth.com

Angela Grassi, MS, RD, LDN

The PCOS Nutrition Center. Specializing in PCOS and distorted eating.

Haverford, PA

www.PCOSnutrition.com

Judy Simon, MS, RD, CD, CHES

Mind Body Nutrition, PLLC. Specializing in nutrition and fertility.

www.mind-body-nutrition.com

Bellevue, WA

Hillary M. Wright, MEd, RD, LDN

Author, freelance writer, consultant. Author, *The PCOS Diet Plan: A Natural Approach to Health for Women with Polycystic Ovary Syndrome* (Ten Speed/Random House, 2010). Director of Nutrition Counseling, Domar Center for Mind Body Health at Boston IVF.

www.pcosdiet.com

hillary@hillarywright.com

Victoria Shanta Retelny, RD, LDN

Writer, speaker, and nutrition communications consultant. Author, *The Essential Guide to Healthy and Healing Foods* (Alpha/Penguin Books, 2011).

www.livingwellcommunications.com

victoria@livingwellcommunications.com

Shivani Sharma, RD, LD, CLT

Specializing in vegetarian diets, IBS, migraine, fibromyalgia and other inflammatory conditions.

Dallas, TX

214-597-6064

shivani@dallasnutritiontherapy.com

www.rightfoodchoice.com

Bridget Swinney, MS, RD

Media representative, Texas Dietetic Association. Author, speaker, spokesperson.

www.healthyfoodzone.com

www.twitter.com/BridgetTxRD

babybitesbook@gmail.com

Heather Neal, RD, LDN

Healthy Glow Prenatal Nutrition. Specializing in trying to conceive and pregnancy nutrition.

336-790-3669

www.healthyglownutrition.com

HeatherRD@nealnutrition.com

Shelley Meyer, D.O., M.S., R.D.

Family physician and registered dietitian, Highlands Health and Wellness.

www.highlandshealthwellness.com

Bonnie Taub-Dix, MA, RD, CDN

Owner, BTD Nutrition Consultants, LLC. Weight loss expert in New York. Author, *Read It Before You Eat It* (Plume). Blogger, *USA Today*:
http://tinuurl.combonnieusatoday

www.betterthandieting.net

Twitter: @eatsmartbd

facebook.com/bonnietaubdix

Dana Angelo White, MS, RD, ATC

Nutrition consultant/certified athletic trainer. Owner, Dana White Nutrition. Nutrition expert for FoodNetwork.com and Healthy Eats blog. Specializing in culinary and sports nutrition.

www.danawhitenutrition.com

www.foodnetwork.com/healthyeats

Bibliography

Books

Chavarro, Jorge E., MD, ScD and Walter C. Willett, MD, DrPH and Patrick J. Skerrett. *The Fertility Diet*. NY: McGraw-Hill, 2008.

D'Adamo, Dr. Peter. J. and Catherine Whitney. *Eat Right For Your Baby*. NY: G.P. Putnam & Sons, 2003.

Murkoff, Heidi and Sharon Mazel. *What To Expect Before You're Expecting*. NY: Workman Publishing Company, Inc., 2009

Ogle, Amy and Lisa Mazzullo, MD. *Before Your Pregnancy*. NY: Ballantine Books/Ballantine Publishing Group, 2002.

Radine Lewis. *The Infertility Cure*. NY: Little, Brown and Company, 2004.

Sterlman, Megan V. *Thinking Pregnant*. Calif: New Harbinger Publications, Inc., 2001.

Tessmer, Kimberly A. *Tell Me What To Eat if I Have Celiac Disease*. Pompton Plains, NJ: Career Press/ New Page Books, 2009.

Online Articles and Websites

The American Congress of Obstetricians and Gynecologists: *www.acog.org*. Accessed October 2010.

"Artificial Sweeteners: Understanding these and other sugar substitutes," from the Mayo Clinic Staff: *http://www.mayoclinic.com/health/artificial-sweeteners/MY00073*. Accessed November 2010.

"Can Your Diet Make You More Fertile?" by Dan Childs: *http://abcnews.go.com/Health/ReproductiveHealth/story?id=4379398&page=1*. Accessed November 2010.

"Certified Organic Label Guide" from Organic.org: *www.organic.org*. Accessed November 2010.

Dietary Guidelines for Americans: *http://www.health.gov/dietaryguidelines*. Accessed October 2010.

"Dietary Reference Intakes for Energy, Carbohydrate, Fiber, Fat, Fatty Acids, Cholesterol, Protein, and Amino Acids", Institute of Medicine of the National Acadamies, http://iom.edu/Reports/2002/Dietary-Reference-Intakes-for-Energy-Carbohydrate-Fiber-Fat-Fatty-Acids-Cholesterol-Protein-and-Amino-Acids.aspx, accessed October 2010.

"8 Ways To Boost Your Fertility," on WebMD: *http://www.webmd.com/baby/guide/8-ways-to-boost-your-fertility*. Accessed October 2010.

Endometriosis.org: *www.endometriosis.org*. Accessed December 2010.

Endo-Online: *www.endo-online.org*. Accessed October 2010.

"Evidence Report of Clinical Guidelines on the Identification, Evaluation, and Treatment of Overweight and Obesity in Adults," MISSING WEBSITE/URL. Accessed October 2010.

"Fats, Carbs and the Science of Conception," from Newsweek. com: *http://www.newsweek.com/2007/12/01/fat-carbs-and-the-science-of-conception.html*. Accessed November 2010.

"Fertility and Diet For Females," from RD411.com: *http://www.rd411.com/index.php?option=com_content&view=article&id=1461:fertility-and-diet-for-females-&catid=100:miscellaneous-topics&Itemid=394*. Accessed October 2010.

"The Full List: 49 Fruits and Veggies" from the Environmental Working Group: *http:/www.foodnews.org/fulllist.php*. Accessed November 2010.

"Getting Pregnant: Understanding Conception," from Baby Med: *www.babymed.com*. Accessed November 2010.

"Getting Pregnant: Ways To Improve Your Fertility," from WebMD: *www.webmd.com*. Accessed November 2010.

"Herbs At A Glance," from National Center for Complimentary and Alternative Medicine: *http://nccam.nih.gov/health/herbsataglance.htm*. Accessed December 2010.

"Herbs at a Glance: A Quick Guide to Herbal Supplements," from NIH, NCCAM, HHS: *http://nccam.nih.gov/health/NIH_Herbs_at_a_Glance.pdf*. Accessed December 2010.

Herbs Research Foundation: *http://www.herbs.org/herbnews/*. Accessed December 2010.

The Hormone Foundation: *www.hormone.org*. Accessed October 2010.

"Infertility and Reproduction Health Center" from WebMD. com: *http://www.webmd.com/infertility-and-reproduction/default.htm*. Accessed October 2010.

Institute of Medicine of the National Academies: *www.iom. edu*. Accessed October 2010.

Natural Medicines Comprehensive Database: *http://naturaldata base. therapeuticresearch.com*. Accessed December 2010.

NIH Office of Dietary Supplements, http://ods.od.nih.gov/, accessed December 2010.

"Omega 3 Fatty Acids During Pregnancy", March Of Dimes, http://www.marchofdimes.com/professionals/ nutrition_omega3more.html, accessed October 2010.

PCOS Nutrition Center: *www.pcosnutrition.com*. Accessed October 2010.

PCOSupport: *www.pcosupport.org*. Accessed October 2010.

"Preconception Health", from Womenshealth.gov, The National Women's Health Information Center: *http:// womenshealth.gov/pregnancy/before-you-get-preg nant/preconception-health.cfm*. Accessed October 2010.

"Pregnancy and Conception," from WebMD: *www.webmd. com/baby/guide/understanding-conception*. Accessed October 2010.

"Recognition and Treatment Approaches For Polycystic Ovary Syndrome," by Angela Grassi, MS, RD, LDN. From Women's Health Dietetic Practice Group: *http://www. womenshealthdpg.org/members/news/Summer_2008. pdf*. Accessed December 2010.

"Treating Infertility Using Acupuncture" from the American Pregnancy Association: *http://www.americanpregnancy. org/infertility/acupunture.htm*. Accessed December 2010.

USDA DRI Tables: *http://fnic.nal.usda.gov/nal_display/index php?info_center=4&tax_level=3&tax_subject= 256&topic_id=1342&level3_id=5140*. Accessed November 2010.

USDA ChooseMyPlate.gov: *www.choosemyplate.gov*. Accessed June 1, 2011.

"Using Dietary Supplements Wisely," from the NIH National Center for Complementary and Alternative Medicine: *http://nccam.nih.gov/health/supplements/wiseuse.htm*. Accessed December 2010.

"What is Reiki?" from the International Center for Reiki Training: *http://www.reiki.org/faq/whatisreiki.html*. Accessed December 2010.

"What You Need to Know about Mercury in Fish and Shellfish," from United States Environmental Protection Agency: *http://water.epa.gov/scitech/swguidance/ fishshellfish/outreach/advice_index.cfm*. Accessed November 2010.

Whole Grains Council: *http://wholegrainscouncil.com/*. Accessed October 2010.

Index

About the Author

Kimberly A. Tessmer, RD, LD, is an author and consulting dietitian in Brunswick, Ohio. Her books include: *The Complete Idiot's Guide to The Mediterranean Diet, Tell Me What to Eat if I Have Celiac Disease, The Everything Nutrition Book,* and *The Everything Pregnancy Nutrition Book.* Kim currently owns and operates Nutrition Focus (*www.nutrifocus.net*), a consulting company specializing in weight management, authoring, menu development, and other nutritional services. In addition, Kim acts as the RD on the board of directors for Lifestyles Technologies, Inc., a company that provides nutrition software solutions, developing a wide array of nutritionally sound menu templates.